The Power
Behind
Your Eyes

The Power
Behind
Your Eyes

Improving Your Eyesight

with Integrated Vision Therapy

by

Robert-Michael Kaplan, O.D., M.Ed.

Healing Arts Press
Rochester, Vermont

Healing Arts Press
One Park Street
Rochester, Vermont 05767
www.InnerTraditions.com

Healing Arts Press is a division of Inner Traditions International

NOTE TO THE READER: This book is intended as an informational guide. The remedies, approaches, and techniques described herein are meant to supplement, and not to be a substitute for, professional medical care or treatment. They should not be used to treat a serious ailment without prior consultation with a qualified healthcare professional.

The information presented in this book is intended to be educational––it is not for diagnosis nor is it a vision-therapy prescription for the treatment of any form of eye condition or disease or any health condition whatsoever. This information should be used to complement a prescribed optometric or ophthalmological vision-care program. The author and publisher are in no way liable for any use or misuse of the contents of this book. The case studies are authentic; however, names and certain details have been changed to protect the identity of these persons.

LIBRARY OF CONGRESS CATALOGING-IN-PUBLICATION DATA
Kaplan, Robert-Michael.
        The power behind your eyes : improving your eyesight with integrated vision therapy / Robert-Michael Kaplan.
            p.   cm.
        Includes bibliographical references and index.
        ISBN 978-0-89281-536-4
        1. Vision disorders—Alternative treatment. 2. Visual training. I. Title.
        RE48.K327   1995
        617.7—dc20   95-24981
                                                                                CIP

Printed and bound in the United States

10 9

Text design and layout by Charlotte Tyler
This book was typeset in Bulmer with Craw Modern as the display typeface

My profound thanks to all of you who, over the years, have contributed to the birth of this book. Lise, my partner in life, whose loving presence, computer skills, and constant encouragement have supported the cocreation of this work. Symon, my son, your smiles open my heart in the morning. Julia, my daughter, for being you. Christopher, your thunderous and compassionate nature inspires my wisdom. Inner Traditions for believing.

May Integrated Vision Therapy reach all those well-deserving souls.

Contents

Foreword   ix

Introduction   1

Chapter 1: The Doorway to Vision   10
  What Is Vision?
  The Anatomy of the Eye
  Eye Symptoms—No Problem

Chapter 2: Opening the Door to the Brain   27
  Storage of Life Experiences
  The Flowing of Our Energy
  Vision and Perception

Chapter 3: Focusing Your Mind   43
  Soul and Personality
  I See with Eye-C Charts
  Cross Your Eyes—They Won't Get Stuck!

Chapter 4: What Do You Want?   60
  Awareness and Healing
  Playing with Resistance
  This Is It
  Surrendering to Fear

Chapter 5: The Challenge to Be Clear   80
  Visual Noise
  Seeing Your Addictions
  Dis-ease Leads to Disease

Chapter 6: What You Say Is What You See!   91
  To Listen Is to Be Liberated
  Victim Vision
  Becoming Empowered through Language

Chapter 7: Your Secret Purpose   105
  Why Are You Here?
  Childhood Dreams
  The Light Within

Chapter 8: Renewing Your Vision   123
  True Self-Expression
  Drastic Intervention
  Seeing Crises Clearly
  Imaging Visual Wellness

Chapter 9: Life's Opportunities   139
  Reclaiming Your Power—Your Naked Vision
  Nearsightedness—Reach Out Fearlessly to the Future
  Farsightedness—Focus Passionately on the Now
  Astigmatism
  Crossed or Wandering Eyes
  What If You Already Have 20/20?
  Eye Diseases—What Can I Do?
  The "Short-Arm" Syndrome—I Am Becoming Wise!
  Help for Your Children's Vision

Chapter 10: Living Your Daily Vision   161

Appendix: The Essential Integrated Vision Therapy Program   169

Bibliography   171
  Suggested Reading
  References

Resources   178

Additional Programs and Services   180

Foreword

D r. Kaplan has written a fascinating and controversial book for the layperson describing in detail the use of vision therapy and nutrition, lifestyle, and attitude changes to improve eyesight. He has found, as have many of us who help people improve their vision, that there is a reciprocal process between insight and eyesight. New insight results from the better vision, and that, in turn, improves eyesight further. These ideas are not as incredible as they sound on first reading. It is becoming increasingly clear in all the medical fields that habits, stress levels, nutritional sins, and the emotional issues of individuals are inextricably related to the quality of their health and outlook. There is no reason to assume that eyes are different from the rest of one's body.

While some people are born with illnesses, including those of the eyes, this should not convince us that all problems are hereditary or that nothing can be done to make changes. In every area people are overcoming acquired and inherited limitations with the help of good healers and teachers. The accounts of patient successes in this book should encourage the reader to take control of his vision by tapping into what Dr. Kaplan calls "the power behind the eyes." Certainly, research supports the idea that amblyopia (lazy eye), much strabismus (crossed or wall eyes), and eye teaming problems can be corrected or improved radically without the risks of surgery. Myopia (nearsightedness) can also be reduced or corrected with vision training.

When I read Dr. Kaplan's manuscript, I was reminded again of my own intense experience giving up nearly all of my nearsightedness over a period of several years in the late 1970s and early 1980s with the help of two behavioral optometrists in Chicago and in Washington, D.C. The results were so stunning that I became an optometrist. My strong lens power (–3.75, the "Big-E-Only" range), which had seemed so necessary before I even dared get out of bed in the morning, was reduced to a –.25 lens. The majority of the lens power was given up by a simple process of gradual lens reduction, faithful wearing of reading glasses weaker than my distance glasses, outdoor distance viewing, good full-spectrum light, optimal nutrition, improved posture, a calm lifestyle, meditation and exercise—all things included in Dr. Kaplan's program. Now, in my own practice, I frequently see new patients who have followed a similar regimen for "other health problems," and then find that their "eyes are hurting" or they "get headaches" wearing their old glasses, which have become too strong. We are immediately able to reduce prescriptions that they apparently needed to see 20/20 prior to the new interest in health and personal development. If more patients and more optometrists were alert to the fact that lens prescriptions can be reduced as well as increased, these changes would be much more commonplace. People need to take charge of their vision, ask for lens reductions, use relaxation techniques prior to exams as Dr. Kaplan suggests, and not make appointments just after school finals, a binge of computer work, or following an illness. Vision can get better gradually, as it once got worse, if people put their minds to it.

To make rapid changes, though, one usually needs actual vision exercises or "vision games," as Dr. Kaplan calls them, and the help of a behavioral optometrist. When one's prescription is finally cut back to the power in the first few pairs of glasses, further change may be more difficult. The process provokes some "looking within," back to the stress patterns that existed when vision started to blur. Most of us went nearsighted when we were too young to analyze our personal stress issues. Since we still needed to see far occasionally, someone sent us off for glasses, which often gave us 20/15 or 20/10 telescopic sight that we confused with good vision. We were able to see the slides from the back of the auditorium without having to recognize that something was amiss that needed a deeper level of fixing. In fact, we were told that our vision was all hereditary and nothing could be done anyway.

If we read through the glasses at all, we increased the strain on our system, which led to "getting worse." The lenses themselves compounded the problem. But the underlying factors such as nutrition, sleep deficits, lifestyle imbalances, excessive computer use, failure to take stock of our needs, and emotional issues that sapped our strength—all went untreated.

There were probably some familial factors of perception style, intensity, focusing ability, and temperament, as well. The lenses substituted for the need to understand our unique problems and inner purposes.

I can remember writing in my journal in 1983 that "myopia does not just drop from the sky or sit bespectacled on the double helix ladder of our genes. It is a choice made, a habit pattern, a mental attitude, I now see." For many people, cutting lens power is as "nonpsychological" as my first two and one half diopters of lens reduction were, but I do not know adults who have dropped close to all the lens power of myopia without noticing some major insights about themselves in youth and childhood, or experiencing some anger or sadness over choices made and the subsequent years of poor vision. One realizes, as Dr. Kaplan suggests, that one has "given one's power away." However, this can be remedied.

After a gradual program to reduce my lens power to the –1.50 range, I began intense in-office training for peripheral vision, for waking up the ambient perceptual system, which is closely connected with posture, balance, awareness, and insight (what Dr. Kaplan calls "retinal vision" as opposed to central or "macular vision"). Soon I could see with less than the lens power in my first pair of glasses. I felt more "in the world," more "face to face." Behind strong lenses, I was behind a barrier. In my weak contacts, the world is more lovely and I am relaxed. Now with my own patients I see that people are more comfortable, more in touch with the world and with themselves when we cut lens power. Both optometrists and patients need to know that lenses allowing 20/15 or even 20/20 crisp acuity in a dark exam room may not be the best standard for good overall vision.

"It is the *phase information,* the volume and complexity, that is lost in the strong lenses," a Harvard post doc said to me that magical day when she could see 20/20 without any lenses. A year earlier she had needed –2.75's.

There is often a continual muscle stress, too, in the neck and around the eyes in strong minus lenses. I believe this is a direct result of placing an oversharpened central image on the fovea (increasing "macular vision") at the expense of the peripheral retina ("retinal vision"). Peripheral vision, when one regains it, gives a startling sense of security in space, better posture, and more relaxed movement.

It is clear to those of us who "went nearsighted" that it is quite an unconscious process, one we can fight against frantically and not be able to stop. We needed the help of informed and skillfully trained optometrists who could have taught us to focus, relax, and coordinate our eyes. Instead, we got what the retinoscope and the phoropter, the autorefractor and our uninformed choices ("Which is better, one or two?") decided was best. The nearsighted adaptation was a useful one in the short run. It allowed us to overuse our vision at near, and narrow our world of attention under stress, so that we could keep going without making any significant changes. It allowed us to get control of a smaller area of our lives—our nearpoint work or study—even as we did not get at the roots of our stresses. We did not have to reassess our nutrition or lifestyle, or pay attention to why we were "zeroing in" and "screening out" and why we had no energy to stay flexible.

In addition to illustrating in detail the concepts I have mentioned, Dr. Kaplan has developed some unique theories about how disruption of good vision happens. He has also had the courage to discuss the mysterious spiritual connection that exists with vision, that goes beyond psychological insights, that opens the "window to the soul." In 1982, I wrote in my journal of vision training that if everyone could see the beauty of the world as I could see it when I first perceived the depth and detail, the volume and intense color that my "strong, old cold lenses" had screened out, "there would be peace on earth because everyone would be too joyous to fight." If I had not written that and other similar perceptions, I might have wondered at Dr. Kaplan's statement that "seeing with your heart means eliminating the pettiness of 'them and us' consciousness." But the fact is, when you can take control of your own vision, use both eyes together, cut lens power, broaden the view—then you are out from behind the glass, back in the world, face to face, one among many, unique in purpose, but connected to all, and you know this in your heart.

Dr. Antonia Orfield, O.D., M.A., FCOVD
Binocular Vision Clinic, The New England Eye Institute
Boston, Massachusetts

Introduction

As you come to recognize the power of your consciousness, what is behind your eyes, so to speak, holds more power than what appears in front of them, your inner and outer perceptions change.

—Gary Zukav

Like millions of others today, you may feel unfulfilled, internally frustrated. Personal computers, cellular telephones, faxes, and electronic kitchen gadgetry may be making your life easier; yet even though you think you have everything, something seems to be missing.

The Power Behind Your Eyes leads you to rediscover that place within that you may have forgotten while building a career, a home, a family. This book focuses on the place inside and around your head and body that remembers the childhood time when life seemed easy and you felt carefree, when days seemed long and each experience was full of excitement. Whether you were running down to the stream, picking wildflowers, playing in the snow, or pirating neighbors' fruits, your vision was filled with multidimensional color. The ever-present thrill of living ran through your body.

This book can awaken in you the power and freedom of a totally drug-free, natural high. *The Power Behind Your Eyes* delves deeply into your perceptions of yourself and the way you perceive life. Your eyes are your primary connection with life. Your perceptions determine the ways you react, make decisions, and conduct your life. By becoming more aware of your current perceptions, you can remove the filtering armor protecting your authentic being and reclaim the natural wisdom you enjoyed as a child.

Power is about being exactly who you are and allowing your innate creative forces to flow. Using that power, you will automatically make career, relationship, and life choices based on new and validated perceptions.

On the surface, this may seem like another esoteric book based on philosophical mumbo jumbo. On the contrary, *The Power Behind Your Eyes* can activate a lifestyle that initiates the self-healing experience through accountable living. As you modify your eyes' perceptive filtering system, you begin to tell the truth about what you see.

The eye is the "satellite dish" of your perceptual (vision) consciousness. The retina of the eye receives light in two ways. A focused beam of light converges onto a specialized part of the retina called the fovea. This is where clear 20/20 vision occurs. I call the mechanics of sight "looking."

On the other hand, when a broad scattering of unfocused light spreads like a paintbrush over the dishlike retina at the back of the eye, blurriness results. This is "seeing." *Looking* at life requires a clear, logical, and analytical process, while *seeing* life means feeling your emotions and intuitively exploring the unknown blurriness.

The Power Behind Your Eyes uses the pragmatic mechanism of your eyes to access your brain and mind. Using specific eye exercises, it is possible to retrain related brain functions and cultivate more effective ways to look *and* see through your eyes. Earlier approaches to better vision were very simplistic and physically oriented. In the 1920s, William Bates, a New York ophthalmologist, proposed that many vision problems developed from overstrain of the muscles surrounding the eyeballs. His remedies were a series of physical exercises, such as covering the eyes with the hands and looking toward the sun. Bates believed this would relax the eye muscles, resulting in clearer eyesight.

The Bates approach has stood the test of time. Some teachers still use this approach from a simpler era, and in some cases it works well despite the complex ways we use our eyes today. However, the modern vision-fitness approach recognizes the intricate connections of all the parts of our being. With our deeper understanding of the workings of the brain, we should incorporate a broader range of techniques to maintain and improve our vision. The physical works alongside the physiological. These processes integrate with the emotional and are influenced by the spiritual aspect of our core nature. *The Power Behind Your Eyes* acknowledges this important holistic connection. The techniques and practices will encourage your brain, mind, and eyes to work together. The Bates system was an important beginning. *The Power Behind Your Eyes* is the next step.

As optometrists diagnosed "problems" and initiated a program of exercises, their patients were able to read more clearly and could look better through their eyes. Vision therapy optometrists then incorporated aspects of psychology and behavior into the treatment. From these new techniques, "patients" increased their self-confidence, children learned more effectively, and eyestrain was controlled.

A science known as behavioral vision therapy has existed for more than twenty years and is now a maturing health discipline that looks at vision from a total-person, or holistic, point of view. (In most of the United States, vision therapy has largely been reimbursed—as much as 80 percent—by major medical coverage.) Behavioral vision therapy has been used to modify both perception and behavior and to provide a dynamic means of becoming "more aware." The most current contribution has been to integrate many medically related disciplines, thus increasing the effectiveness of vision therapy as a total healing system. Scientific research has confirmed the clinical discoveries of Integrated Vision Therapy. Its premise is that through the eyes, we now have the ability to change our physical well-being and the way we behave. Our behavior can either stem from the ego-driven state, "looking"—that is, what we believe to be our inherent makeup, our personality—or be more heart connected, where aspects of our soul are expressed. Life becomes an opportunity to discover the balance and harmony between the body, mind, and eye states.

"The eyes are the window to the soul," Shakespeare said. Those of us who have been told we need eyeglasses to see best can discover what our eyes and mind are attempting to reveal to us. Our lens prescription provides the clues we need.

Like most optometrists, I once thought having my patients wear a compensating lens prescription over their eyes would solve their problems. I remember exactly when my way of looking at my patients' vision problems changed for me. I was sitting in my cubbyhole of an office in Durban, South Africa. My typical day was spent in this dark room, hardly seeing my patients because of the lack of light, and saying, "Is it better with lens one or lens two? Now, is it better with one or two?"

One day I sat back in my office chair, pulled away that funny machine we eye doctors put in front of your eyes to keep ourselves from really connecting (I learned this part later), and looked into my patient's eyes. For the first time, I really joined with the human being sitting there with me. I felt a thrill of joy move through my heart. Reaching out, I gently touched my patient's hands and said, "I really want to help you see and not have you become addicted to these eyeglasses." As I spoke, tears welled up in her eyes.

For a moment, I sat tilting backward in my chair. Many thoughts flashed through my mind. Was I willing to say, "Is it better with one or two?" for the rest of my life, ninety-three times a day, five days a week, forty-nine weeks a year, for another forty years? Surely, there was something more empowering for me to share with my patients.

I studied my patient's measured prescription—farsightedness with astigmatism—and remembered how we were taught in optometry school to make a diagram of the prescription. I quickly drew a diagram of the prescription on a piece of paper and noticed there was more blurring in the vertical part of the astigmatic orientation than the horizontal. I looked at the patient and realized that her body, like the astigmatism, could also be thought of as comprising both a vertical component (upright head to toes) and a horizontal one (outstretched arms from right to left). Perhaps, I mused, the measured optical prescription is a spatial map of how the patient organizes her visual and body space.

I became very excited with this concept, and my daily "ones and twos" took on a new meaning. I began talking more with my patients. Soon after this experience, an optometric colleague suggested that he begin administering vision therapy on *me*. I jumped at the opportunity. As I mastered the techniques, I began teaching the vision games (as I call them) to my patients, in a brightly lit room, with no "ones or twos."

As the patients integrated the new therapy, I noticed a peculiar phenomenon. The previous rigid eye measurements of the patients were now becoming more variable. This confused me at first. When I asked patients how they felt about their vision, they reported more flexibility and freedom in their perceptions of their lives. I began to appreciate how, as a vision therapist, I could access the patients' minds through their eyes and bring about perceptual changes. I continued modifying their lens prescriptions to weaker and weaker configurations, so my patients were increasingly challenged to deal with their visual blocks and limited perceptions. As they began to claim more of the power behind their eyes, their self-image and their outlook began to change.

Using Eastern methods of analysis, Ayurvedic medicine, and my own experience with the South African nativistic rituals, I began viewing the left eye as the "feminine channel" and the right as the "masculine channel." The perceptual correlates of *looking*—the rational, intellectual, and analytical characteristics—matched the right-eye perceptions quite well; the perceptual correlates of *seeing*—the creative, intuitive, and nonlinear characteristics—matched the left eye. However, I remained cognizant of the multiple crossovers of the neurological pathways of either eye to both hemispheres.

Like a fingerprint, each lens prescription is different. The degree of farsightedness (clearer perception at far distances) or nearsightedness (clearer perception close up) reflects how we deal with our world or personal space. Nearsightedness is an accumulation of mind misperceptions that are constrictive in nature. Your eyes have been programmed by your mind to see the world as being closer than it really is. This way of looking is overly focused and inner directed. Farsightedness is a mental encoding that claims that your view of life is expansive and broad. Through your inaccurate perceptions you believe the world to be farther away than it really is. Farsightedness programming of your eyes means that you prefer to look ahead and deal with the future rather than the now.

Astigmatism is an unequal curvature or warpage of the cornea. It is an external printout of rigidity in perception. This perceptual distortion is a reaction to a non-presence in one or more parts of your life. Astigmatism is a perceptual discord between your genetic reality and the way you have chosen to view your current life experiences. The belief system built around these perceptions is one of feeling as if you don't fit in. The most common variety of astigmatism is related to avoidance of being aligned with your soul truth. Through these eye conditions, or messages from the eye/brain, you can determine which areas of your "life" perceptions are more distorted than others.

The process of opening perceptions through vision games seemed simple. But with deeper investigation, I became aware of how the lens prescription measurements could vary between the right and left eyes. Why did people present such varying perceptions?

Whether or not you need to wear corrective lenses, the way you use each eye tells a remarkable story about your perceptions in relationships, career, and creative endeavors. Our earliest stimulation and development of perceptions is derived from our interactions with our parents. The blueprint for these perceptions is coded at conception from the genes of our mother and father. Extrapolating from Denny Johnson's Rayid model of iris interpretation as well as the fields of genetics and family tree origins, I came to believe that the right eye perceptions follow the DNA code of our father's side of the family, and the left eye perceptions, our mother's. This perceptual unfolding, predisposed from the genetic DNA material, is further influenced by our life experiences. For example, we may carry a hereditary trait of predisposition toward anger from our father, and if, in our early experiences, he models this anger for us, we have two clear messages about how to be angry—one from the genetic predisposition and one based on his modeling. According to the Rayid model, over forty such influences can be passed down through the four generations preceding ours. These DNA-transmitted behavioral predispositions influence our perceptions, our vision choices, and the adaptations we make.

In Japanese macrobiotics, the universe is defined in an orderly Yin and Yang form. These divisions are energy forms. Ideally, they interact equally with each other, providing a dynamic and balanced energy state. Yin energy is expansive, peripheral, and female and involves space. Yang energy is contracting, central, male, and time-based. The right eye, then, is equivalent to Yang-based energy—expressive, male, outward-perceiving. The left eye, Yin-based, is receptive and female, with inward-based perceptions. Vision through the right eye reveals aspects of personality and behavior associated with the father's side of the family. I call this perception "Harry." "Sally" refers to the perceptions of the left eye, influences and factors affecting vision from the mother's side of the family.

My first clinical visual therapy experiment was performed while my patients covered one eye and then spoke about their feelings, experiences, and emotional responses. I noticed that when the left eye was covered, the communication was generally more rational, focused, and linear. With the right eye covered, the expressive style was emotional, feeling, and creative. These behaviors replicated what research has revealed about brain function; that is, the left brain engages more in analytical thinking, while the right brain is employed for intuitive, creative ways of being. From an energetic point of view, I extrapolated that the right eye could be considered a male/left-brain equivalent, and the left eye a female/right-brain equivalent. The Rayid method of iris interpretation corroborated my theory by implicating the right iris as carrying the genealogical patterns of the father's side of the family and the left iris as carrying the mother's. I then related this data to the Yin and Yang connections as described in the principles of macrobiotics. The process of developing my work in visual therapy was an evolutionary one, each phase being a building block for the next. Later, my exploration of spirituality in the Jewish Kabbalah and Tibetan Buddhist traditions brought into focus the mind's (as opposed to the brain's) relationship to vision. The idea that we misperceive the reality of the world became the area of my clinical investigations. My intuitive African heritage, based on a perceptual style of seeing life from a standpoint of interrelatedness and holism, helped me to integrate many disciplines and experiences that built a case for the model of holistic integrated vision therapy. My patients, numbering in the tens of thousands, helped me recognize these connections, while my ongoing personal experiment with double vision gave me incredible insights into what vision really is.

As we evolve we integrate both the receptive and the expressive vision styles. At any point, however, this process of integration can be interrupted, and one of those perceptual channels can end up dominating our vision of life. When one eye dominates in vision more than the other and results in a predominant way of looking, such as having too much central focus, this predominance can turn into nearsightedness or astigmatism for that particular eye. On the other hand, if the perception through one eye is too expansive, or too much of the retina is being stimulated, then this may result in farsightedness, which ultimately can be measured in that eye. If we are looking more through either Harry or Sally, we may be programming an incomplete perceptual experience into our consciousness.

I believe that when the dominant perception comes through the left eye, our view of life will be more Yin—more creative and emotional—and be either limited or expansive depending upon the perceptions passed down genealogically from our mother. The opposite is true for right-eye domination. Our vision of life is more rational and focused and influenced by the beliefs and perceptions learned or modeled after our father and his side of the family. Ideally, the two perceptions integrate in what Carl Jung called the "divine marriage."

When the left and right eye states are balanced and integrated, we are able to see in a multidimensional fashion. In conventional vision therapy this is called binocular stereoscopic vision. According to Gary Zukav, author of *The Seat of The Soul*, "The perceptions of a multisensory human extend beyond physical reality to the larger dynamical systems of which our physical reality is a part. The multisensory human is able to perceive, and to appreciate, the role that our physical reality plays in the larger picture of evolution, and the dynamics by which our physical reality is created and sustained. This realm is invisible to the five-sensory human."

From an eyesight and vision point of view, this dimension of vision, beyond the sensory state, probably includes the soul. When we limit our perceptions to just the senses, are we focusing through the eyes of personality? If this is true, then in visual terms, are we limiting our potential, as we dominate our looking through either Harry or Sally? I do know that when one of these perceptions has more control than the other, we are imbalanced and feel incomplete. In Integrated Vision Therapy, the enhancement of eyesight includes our becoming aware of vision beyond the physical sense of sight—vision that permits us to look into the invisible. This form of seeing is accessing the power behind our eyes.

The Power Behind Your Eyes is not a book intended to help you become more industrious in the way you are *doing* things in your life. The awareness we seek has to do with *being*. The eyes are only the doorway to your vision. The meaning of *vision* goes beyond how clearly you see, extending to the way you experience your self-image, aspirations, fears, and family ties. Sometimes, unbeknown to you, the choices you make today are being negatively influenced by earlier events in your life or the lives of your parents or grandparents. These inherited influences, subtle though they may be, steer you away from your own real purpose. Through increasing your awareness, *The Power Behind Your Eyes* can help you discover why you behave the way you do, and further presents the option of "living your vision," making new life choices with clarity and awareness. The primary purpose of this book is to inspire you to begin this journey into the discovery of your true potential through the doorway of your eyes.

I began exploring vision therapy twenty years ago. My initial investigations were conducted in the clinical practice of optometry. I then joined the faculty of optometry at the University of Houston, where I taught vision therapy and pursued clinical studies of how the two eyes work in unison. During this time I became a vegetarian and noticed how my own double vision seemed less predominant. I later began modifying lens prescriptions in an attempt to keep my patients from relying on ever-stronger eyeglasses. At the same time I was studying visual science in a graduate degree program in physiological optics and was there exposed to basic research on visual function. This study formed the basis for such therapeutic interventions as covering one eye with a patch as a way to retrain brain functioning. Growing bored with basic research, I soon expanded my master's degree work to include studies in education and psychology, at which time I learned how perceptions are formed and how malleable the brain really is. I worked with children who were both physically handicapped and visually and/or auditorally impaired. With patience and therapeutic ingenuity, I saw children with severe developmental handicaps begin to gain mastery of their bodies and brain functions. Integrated vision therapy grew out of these experiences, supported by my intuitive African Jewish heritage.

The major portion of the information I'll be sharing with you in this book reflects my personal journey and my own research into the connection between the mind, brain, body, and eyes.

My presentation of this advanced, state-of-the-art method is more experiential than simply knowledge-oriented. An important new model for learning is a nonintellectual, knowledge-based approach that takes place in the relaxed, creative alpha cycle of the brainwave patterns. Instead of "trying to understand," you can receive information and process it in your higher brain centers through awareness. The applications of this model can be immediately useful in your daily life. Practical activities are included in this book so you can experiment on your own.

The power behind the eyes is the inner wisdom that already exists in each one of us. Removing the camouflage nets that cover the hidden places within our existence gives us the opportunity to set our perceptions free. We can open our eyes to *see* what we really *feel* is of value in our lives, instead of what we may *think* is important.

The Power Behind Your Eyes offers an opportunity for the unification of all parts of your being. The message is quite simple. There is nothing you must do, other than *be*.

Chapter 1

The Doorway to Vision

What Is Vision?

If I were to ask you what vision means, you might say it is how accurately you see, how sharp your eyesight is, or possibly how well you see a perfect 20/20 on an eye chart. Others might understand vision to be esoteric insights from the mind. All these definitions are valid.

We have been programmed to believe the eye is like a camera that captures an image on a film equivalent, the retina. In reality, however, your eyes merely *contribute* to your vision; they are the doorway to your mind. They receive and organize light and then dispense that light, which sets in motion the transfer of energy to the understanding mind, which then constructs the experience of what you perceive and see. These incredible organs are microcosms of your whole body. The light interacts with live tissue, and the combined energy is fed to your brain, where 90 percent of the process we call "vision" occurs. Yet, most optometrists (vision doctors specializing in diagnosing vision disturbances) and ophthalmologists (medical doctors specializing in eye diseases) determine the quality of your vision by examining only your eyes themselves. Their professional focus has been on the disease process, or on what's wrong with the way you *look*.

The unfortunate reality is that during routine eye examinations, most assessments focus on checking only the quality of eye health rather than the effectiveness of your individual capacity to organize and process incoming light. Why don't most eye doctors consider other aspects of the person?

This style of practice is modeled around a medical-insurance system that reimburses payment to the attending professional when a physical problem is discovered, and thus encourages discovery of such problems. Patients, however, often pursue cases of false diagnosis, and ultimately the lucrative industry of malpractice suits has become a giant threat to health-care professionals.

Vision-care professionals, like most medical doctors, have responded to this threat by implementing more and more tests for their patients, to ensure the identification of any possible eye diseases. The initial idea of prevention was good, but the situation reached paranoid proportions in the mid-1980s, when 80 to 90 percent of the total time allotted for an eye-vision examination was devoted to a search for the presence of eye disease. Only 10 to 20 percent of the assessment time considered how well the eyes worked and how well they were able to convey information from the eye to the brain. Only a small minority of eye doctors, possibly 15 percent (mostly progressive vision therapy or behavioral optometrists), ventured into seeing the patient as a person with eyes. These behaviorally trained optometrists are skilled in examining vision from a functional and enhancement point of view. But just look in the Yellow Pages to note how many ophthalmologists limit their practices to the retina or the cornea or to a specialty in microsurgery.

When optometrists advertise their services, they often seem to highlight their fashion-frame selection. In the 1980s, consumerism reached its maturity in North America. The vision-care industry focused on the mass marketing of eyewear products because it seemed more money could be made by selling eyeglasses or contact lenses than through preventative vision care. Some of the corporate giants in cosmetics and pharmaceuticals took contact lenses under their product wings. Designer-frame manufacturers also got in on the action, preying on vanity-conscious eyeglass wearers.

This end-product approach to eye care has overshadowed the emphasis on vision. Less money is invested in the vision examination than in the vision-care products (eyeglasses, contact lenses, solutions, medications, and the like). As consumers, our thinking about vision has been relegated to the physical plane of getting our vision back to 20/20. *The Power Behind Your Eyes* suggests a fresh and empowering way of seeing vision and the care and maintenance of our eyes.

Vision is a process, a dynamic state of doing and being. "Doing" is associated with the rational and logical day-to-day existence of busy-ness and accomplishing tasks. "Being" is the time out, the relaxing, the letting go, the kicking back from the busy-ness of life. Ideally, these two behavioral states interweave to produce a physiological dance that harmonizes our internal organs, muscles, and, most importantly, our nervous system.

For most of us, this dance is not occurring in balanced measure. For the majority of people, "doing" dominates daily existence. An astute vision therapy optometrist (a doctor who prescribes eyeglasses from a conservative and therapeutic point of view and who offers special exercises for enhancing vision) can measure deviations from the norm in your eyes and can interpret the relationship between these measurements and the way you use your vision in life.

Clinical research tells us that the eye responds to most of the physiological processes of the body. The nervous system that warns you to slam on the brakes of your car is routed through your eyes; the sugar processed through your pancreas affects the way you focus; a stimulating landscape modifies the size of your pupils. A larger pupil reflects the fight-or-flight response, and a smaller pupil indicates a relaxed state. Learning as much as possible about visual function can help you make healthy life choices and help you teach your children how to have integrated, powerful, and clear vision as they get older.

I was once afflicted by double vision during 50 percent of my waking hours. In spite of clear eyesight and perfect 20/20 vision, when I was looking far away or attempting to read, two images of the scene would suddenly appear. Have you ever tried dealing with two sets of headlights hurtling down the freeway toward you? (I recall driving Interstate 5, south of Seattle, when my double vision contributed to the arrival of my car and me in the center highway ditch.) Try reading what appears to be two books at the same time. It is very disconcerting. (Not surprisingly, I chose the path of being a non-reader.)

The times when I wasn't seeing double generally were times when I felt relaxed. My double vision taught me that I needed to focus my attention more in order to be present and single in my vision. It was easy for me to "space out." My double vision seemed to increase with the amount of distress I experienced when I worked long hours; it also increased when I ingested refined, fatty foods and when I deprived my body of sufficient sleep, fresh air, and exercise. These variables affected my ability to stay focused and present and encouraged me to "space out." As children, the importance of these elements to a healthy life is drummed into us and we, in turn, preach it to our children. But sometimes we forget. When I realized that lack of exercise, for example, was affecting my vision and my state of well-being, I woke up to the need to modify my unhealthy lifestyle.

I also discovered an emotional connection to my vision. Each time my father, who lived abroad, visited me, I had episodes of double vision. Our relationship has always been rather turbulent, and when reacting to him, I would experience dramatic changes in my vision. My patients have reported similar changes in vision: negative, fearful, or angry thoughts and limiting beliefs seem to cause increased blurring. In his book *And There Was Light*, Jacques Lusseyran talks of being blind at the age of eight and of his subsequent recovery process. In the beginning, he was able to experience the full richness of nonreflected light within his eyeball only when he could free his mind of limiting thoughts, self-pity, and other self-defeating perceptions.

In my case, after undergoing specific vision therapy exercises and routines, I developed the ability to use my brain to control my eye muscles. The periods of double vision diminished, but not completely, because I still hadn't learned how to control my limiting thoughts and fears. Certainly the prismatic lenses in my eyeglasses helped me maintain single vision, but when I took them off, my double vision became worse. Only when I used the full, mind-controlled vision, seeing through *both* my eyes, did I understand that the patterns of my unconscious perceptions caused blurry and double vision to surface.

The Anatomy of the Eye

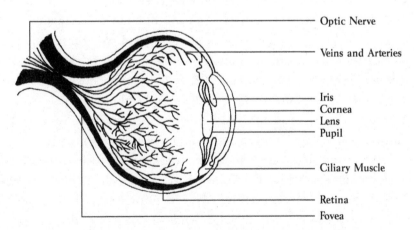

© 1994 From the book Seeing Without Glasses. Beyond Words Publishing Inc. Hillsboro, Or. Used with permission.

- Almost 50 percent of the cranial nerves that emanate from the brain and control all bodily functions are for the specific use of the eyes.
- Some structures in the eye function without a direct blood supply of their own.
- The internal lens of the eye, which is like a transparent windowpane, has its own metabolic system for regenerating cells.
- The outer surface of the eye (the anterior layer of the cornea) can regenerate itself in twenty-four hours.

The retina has two structures, rods and cones. The cones are used for daytime vision (most of the cones are in the macula and fovea area, the place for 20/20 central sight), and the rods are for night vision. Another aspect of the way our eyes work, which most non-vision therapy eye doctors don't really consider, is that the fovea and retina of one eye have to collaborate with the fovea and retina of the other eye. The thoughts, feelings, and emotions we experience through these eye structures influence our perceptions of life, and most of the decisions we make—as well as the ways we play sports, are drawn to careers, hobbies, and mates, and use our vision—are influenced by these inner perceptions.

You may be one of the millions who have excellent 20/20 eyesight. However, perhaps you cannot concentrate efficiently for more than thirty minutes of reading, working at a computer, or sewing, for instance, without having your mind wander, forgetting what you just read, or feeling pain in your eyes. If that is the case, the right fovea and retina are not cooperating with the left fovea and retina. They're having a fight; they're dysfunctional together.

Clear 20/20 eyesight is achieved through the fovea, which metaphorically represents clarity, focus, detail, logic, precision, rationality, and analysis. The foveal qualities of perception are culturally associated with a *doing* mode. The peripheral retina relates to *being* and represents feelings, emotions, creativity, sensing, and intuition. In my earlier book, *Seeing Without Glasses* (formerly *Seeing Beyond 20/20*), I termed the foveal, or *doing*, process "looking" and the working of the peripheral retina, the *being* process, "seeing." The terms are borrowed from the great teacher Frederick Franck, who, in *The Zen of Seeing*, teaches an innovative drawing process.

While studying with Franck for a weekend, my wife and I found ourselves looking at leaves. Dr. Franck had us draw their physical details—a very demanding visual exercise. We had to remember to breathe and let our eyes scan every inch of the leaf while our fingers guided our pens over the sketchbook page. The representation was amazing. But an element was missing: *seeing* the leaf. Without allowing the emotion and feeling through the retina to also be involved in the drawing, it became too technically perfect and lacked warmth and heartfelt connection.

Through the retina, we feel and sense emotions and open up another form of awareness triggered by movement and blurring. This may come as a surprise. *Seeing* with the retina reveals double and blurry vision perceptions. The more we could remain aware of the blurring, or "ground," around the edges of the leaf, the more *life* we were able to put into the leaf drawing.

After I finally gave up the disciplined *looking* mode of my formal education, I came to describe the combination of *looking* and *seeing* as a process called Integrated Vision. The power behind your eyes is a way of using your eyes in which you become simultaneously aware of what is in front of you as well as what is on the side (peripheral seeing). My own double vision, for instance, had actually been activated in my mind through a combination of hereditary factors and life experiences. Without *looking* directly at my father or mother, that is, by only focusing behind them in a farsighted way, I was only *seeing* them, which created the double vision. I learned that this kind of vision was physiologically acceptable and emotionally contained. When I experienced blurry and double vision, I would bring forth my new power, which was the ability to focus close and inward. When I integrated my looking and seeing, my double vision experiences occurred less than 3 percent of the time. Within six months, I didn't need prismatic prescription glasses anymore. I was set free.

Now in my forties, I still have excellent eyesight for reading, yet I have been warned repeatedly by my colleagues that inevitably I will need reading glasses because of the cursed "short-arm" syndrome—someday, they say, my arm will not be long enough to bring details into focus by moving an object farther away. What I haven't told them is that I practice my Integrated Vision Therapy daily and intend to do so forever, just as I brush my hair and floss my teeth. My vision is well worth the few extra minutes a day.

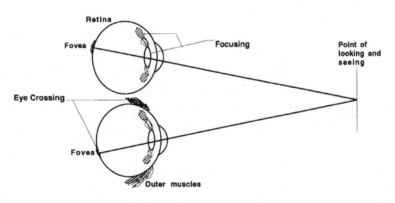

FOCUSING
AND CLARITY

FOCUSING is asking the question: *"What is it you see?"*
(This is dealing with blur.)

EYE CROSSING is asking the question: *"Where is it, what you see?"*
(This is dealing with single vision.)

Control + Power = Clarity

Control − Power = Survival (This is called BLUR.)

Focusing (Clarity) + Eye Crossing = Integrated TWO-EYEDNESS
(Multidimensional vision)

15

When we were kids, my brother and I had an old projector lens that magnified the details of our stamp collection. One sunny day we were playing outside. To our delight, we found that when we focused sunlight through the lens onto a piece of paper, the page started to burn. Similarly, an eyeglass or contact lens focuses light fiercely onto the fovea on the retina at the back of the eye. This explosion of light causes an overstimulation of foveal energy at the expense of retinal function. This means most lens prescriptions cause more *doing* and *looking* in our lives, and less *being* or *seeing*. Is it possible that our perceptions are influenced by the way strong 20/20 eyeglasses and contact lenses focus light to the fovea? It's horrific to think, for example, that workaholism may be encouraged by the artificial lenses we look through.

In the United States alone, 132 million people wear eyeglasses and contact lenses. Twenty-five percent of the world's population is nearsighted. If something seems wrong with our eyes, we often give away our power of choice to the optometrist or ophthalmologist and he or she substitutes an artificial power in the form of a lens prescription. Eyeglasses or contacts replace our innate power (the power behind our eyes), and we become dependent on an outside source of power. That outside source of power becomes a crutch.

I felt compelled to experiment with different lens prescriptions to see if behavior indeed changed when the light through the eyes was more widely dispersed over the retina and not just concentrated over the fovea. What I ultimately observed, over twenty years of clinical investigation, seems to support my hypothesis: not only do weaker lens prescriptions encourage more seeing than looking, they create the perfect biofeedback mechanism for you to observe your thoughts, emotions, and feelings. This witnessing process helps you be aware that the blurring of your seeing can fluctuate in certain circumstances. This process will be explained in more detail shortly.

This connection between eyesight and emotion is the future of vision care. It is available to you now if you are willing to commit to being an active participant in your personal healing journey.

Eye Symptoms—No Problem

My friend in Oregon drives a BMW—a sleek and technologically sophisticated automobile. One day while driving with him, I noticed some black tape covering a flashing red light on the dash. "Dick, what does this light mean? Why is it flashing?" I asked. He replied, "Oh, that's just to let me know I need to service the engine. I have about three thousand kilometers left before I really need to do anything about it."

For a moment I thought how strange it was that he would question German technology. The light was on because something needed to be checked in the engine, and here he was covering up the light. How much in denial are we about what's really happening to us? How often do we just cover up our symptoms, the blurring of our life? How often do we try to cover up these symptoms that could help us wake up and perceive?

The example of the red light made me curious. I began to look at my own eye and body symptoms and at every little message transmitted by my body. I recall a profound conversation with my daughter when I felt an incredible pain in the right side of my head as she talked about her life with me. As she shared her feelings, my pain seemed to fluctuate. Before I had begun to notice the messages my body was sending me, I probably wouldn't have paid much attention to the pain—I wouldn't have been that aware. But in this moment, I happened to be tuning in. I felt my chest becoming very tight. I was beginning to shut down and to feel anger and frustration. I seized the moment and, with it, the opportunity to face my own fears of rejection and losing love.

With an honest assessment of our particular needs and fears, and with clarity of mind, we can begin to understand that physical symptoms are revealing something very important. I began to talk to my patients about vision with the understanding that important information was being communicated from their minds through their eye conditions.

When you think about it, an optometrist or an ophthalmologist usually doesn't bear good news. Focusing on the projected eye chart may bring forth fearful memories of when your doctor told you you needed eyeglasses, contacts, medications, or surgery. By and large, our relationship with eye-care professionals is based on the assumption that our eyes will fail us. The first step in changing vision, however, is to modify limiting perceptions. Symptoms such as blurring, double vision, red eyes, pain in the eyes, gritty or sandy sensations, and diagnosed conditions such as glaucoma, cataracts, and astigmatism can be viewed as good news.

For most of my patients (and for me), this change of attitude required a quantum leap to a new way of thinking. How could a blinding and potentially life-challenging disease like glaucoma be viewed as a gift? But consider this computer analogy: if 90 percent of vision is initiated from the mind, then isn't it possible that the eye is like a printout that helps us understand our inner thinking, our mind's perceptions? I concluded that the conditions I measured in the eye and the ways of looking and seeing through

Harry and Sally, as well as the way they interact, are like a faxed message from your perceptual consciousness. Deep inside your subconscious, a little voice is calling you to action. "Your lifestyle is out of balance, too much *doing* (or *being*) is happening. I am going to send a message, an eye condition like nearsightedness (or glaucoma or astigmatism), to wake you up to this imbalance and abuse."

Your eyes are like the red warning light on my friend's car. You can choose to ignore the wake-up call, but eventually you'll have to deal with the consequences, such as further deterioration of your eyesight or loss of the maximum use of your eyes. On the other hand, you can acknowledge the sensitive reporting system of your eyes and say, "Thank you, my beautiful eyes, for letting me know I need to do something different here."

When I was teaching vision therapy in a college of optometry at Pacific University in Portland, Oregon, I shared this innovative concept with a patient. Unlike the strange looks I usually received, this young woman's reaction told me she immediately understood my line of reasoning. "You mean," she said, "my mind is trying to tell me something through my eyes?" During two subsequent office visits, we determined that her loss of sharp vision for distances (nearsightedness) correlated with her having started an intense course of studies at the university. She needed to adjust her vision to constant close-up focus for reading many books. Without a relaxing program in place for her eyes and vision, extensive reading was not in the best interests of her eyes, body, and mind.

Our eyes are still biologically designed for hunting and farming. When we read, our mind is focused on absorbing information, making good grades, or perhaps accomplishing our career objectives. Our mind says to our eyes, "Please stay focused and look clearly at the little words on the page." Over time, this strong, close-up communication of eye to page leaves the focusing muscle inflexible and thus unable to relax when looking far away. Blurry eyesight results.

Before, when you thought something was wrong with your eyes, you ran to the eye doctor for a solution. The bad news was that you needed glasses to "correct your problem." This is further from the truth than the nearest star is from our planet. In my research, the long-term use of traditional, "corrective" 20/20 lenses leads to further reductions in eyesight. Other contributing factors to vision's becoming even more blurry are excessive reading, lack of sleep, or eating foods that set up an allergic metabolic reaction.

I began experimenting with weaker lens prescriptions for 20/40. Instead of using 20/20—that is, instead of neutralizing the blur to zero—I left about 16 percent in place, which resulted in 84 percent clearness. Accompanied by vision therapy, this practice gave my patients a therapeutic edge. If my patients conscientiously followed my home-based Integrated Vision Therapy program for increasing vision fitness in both eyes, and if they learned how to integrate these perceptions, they eventually were able to use even weaker lens prescriptions. Over time, the 16 percent blur actually lessened. This was true corrective lens prescribing.

In the late 1970s and early 1980s, as a professor of clinical optometry encouraged to do research I was in a very fortunate position. I could delve into the possibilities of new information that would further advance the science of vision. In recording the responses of clinical trials, I noted that as my patients reported their eye symptoms a story emerged that correlated particular events in their life with their eyes and vision. An implied metaphoric truth began to surface. I also discovered that like my patient's stories, each part of the eye's anatomy reflected pieces of its own story about vision, communicating specific needs coming from the mind—needs wanting acknowledgment and action.

For example, I found that a symptom and subsequent diagnosis related to the cornea of the eye, with indications such as pain, a breakdown of the integrity of the tissue, or inflammation, correlated to aspects of a power struggle in the person's life. The cornea of the eye contributes at least 80 percent of the optical refraction of light that ultimately reaches the fovea. If you look at the cornea in cross section, you see an exquisite structure, beautifully shaped, totally transparent, like a clear dome. When we become perceptually unconscious, the natural functions of the parts of the eye become threatened with warpage and distortion. The cornea covers the iris, the colored part of the eye. When the dome is warped so that the refractive capacity of the cornea is stronger in one location than another, the condition of astigmatism exists.

To be able to acknowledge pain and discomfort in the presence of problematic diagnoses and to still see the light at the end of the tunnel is a challenge for anyone. It takes honestly finding a place deep within the essence of who we are to be able to see past the hurdle. This kind of powerful seeing comes from spirit or the soul. Gary Zukav says this in *The Seat of The Soul:* "When we see through authentically powered eyes, metaphorically speaking, one has more ability to see without obstruction, more ability to live love and wisdom, and more ability and desire to help others evolve into the same love and light." I believe that with Integrated Vision Therapy we can extend this idea beyond the metaphor. The power behind our eyes is the acknowledgment of an energy larger than just the presence of our eyes. This essence, or soul, contributes to our having clear vision, which in turn stimulates our eyes to function well.

Stephen At age twenty-two, Stephen had been enticed by catchy advertisements for corneal laser surgery that would correct his nearsightedness once and for all. He could see with perfect 20/20 vision using his eyeglasses, and with a great degree of comfort. The seduction of the surgery was the promise of freedom from nearsightedness and from the need to wear glasses.

He made what he thought were the necessary educated investigations into this experimental procedure. Stephen was told that a minimum number of symptoms would result from the surgery and, with time and healing, they would all go away. He went ahead with the laser surgery. The first procedure on the right eye was only partially successful; a second procedure was later required on the same eye. But the physician was elated by Stephen's technically perfect 20/20 vision without glasses.

At first, the novelty of looking clearly without glasses blinded him to the minor irritation and symptoms of cloudy perception. As the weeks and months went by and he waited for the corneal tissue to continue healing, he slipped into depression. Formerly an outgoing young man with lots of friends, he became more introverted, stayed at home, and went back to living with his mother. His successful career seemed purposeless. He became unemployed and spent hours at home, just sitting around moping. His friends and mother couldn't understand what was happening to him.

About that time, he consulted with me. I was flabbergasted when, in a subdued voice, he shared his main concern. I quote: "I don't want to be looking through these eyes." His choice of an invasive surgical approach to enhance his vision, and this profound comment, reveal how Stephen had disconnected himself from his eyes.

Stephen also mentioned that although his corneas had healed, a floater (matter in the vitreous jelly of the eye) was annoying him. Even though Stephen had clear 20/20 vision without glasses, the presence of the floater and his cloudy vision destroyed all the benefits of the surgery. What was this message from Stephen's unconscious mind? Why was this symptom such bad news for this man? Could I assist him in discovering the good news in such a relatively nonreversible eye condition as a floater? Had the floater always been present and had the corneal laser surgery simply magnified the condition? Was the floater a result of surgical trauma?

I couldn't answer all these questions, but I could assist Stephen by looking at the eyes' message. A big, underlying question still loomed. Was

Stephen ready to step out of his "victim" shoes and begin to take responsibility for his own vision of life?

As is the case with many of my patients, Stephen and I covered a lot of ground during his first visit. He discovered how his eyes could influence many aspects of his life. His most important realization was that he feared making further medical decisions about his eyes in case there would once again be negative consequences. The fear, which first occurred when his original doctor diagnosed his nearsightedness, had really never been dealt with.

Stephen took a year to ponder the outcome of our first meeting—and then he unexpectedly phoned. I knew he had gained deep insights. At his second consultation, Stephen's attitude seemed different. He appeared more comfortable with the bad news of his predicament, even though the eye symptoms had only vaguely subsided. He spoke with more assurance and personal ownership of his eye difficulties. Rather than blaming the experience, he seemed to be taking charge of the circumstances of his life. This is not uncommon in true healing that is soul-driven. Stephen had to see the purpose of his condition and kindle his intention to become well through modification of his lifestyle.

By integrating the emotional experiences revealed through his eyes, Stephen began to make prudent life choices. This created the context for later physical treatments to heal the floaters and discomfort he felt in the eyes themselves.

Cases like Stephen's are not unique. If the premise is that vision begins in the mind and that our eye symptoms and vision distortions are present to wake us up, then perhaps the waking-up process needs to be gradual. Perhaps the message here is that we should see life as a journey, savoring every moment rather than being overfocused on the close-up destination. A process like the corneal laser technique is very quick. The mind has little time to prepare for the return of such sharp degrees of vision. The symptoms that frequently result after eye surgery might be translated as the mind screaming out for attention. "You didn't get the message the first time, so now I *really* need to emphasize it!"

Quite often, my patients have a specific eye condition and are trying to mask the messages that are coming through. The condition may go away, and in many cases it stays away for awhile. Then wham!—a second symptom or condition manifests itself. With the more gradual approach of using weaker and weaker lens prescriptions, coupled with specific Integrated

Vision Therapy, the brain and the mind seem to have a more reasonable opportunity to accommodate the new vision.

Integrated Vision Therapy is like building a house. The foundation needs to be sturdy in order to support the other structures. You are on a journey of discovery, and each stage of the journey needs to be fully embraced and accepted in its time. You see the general picture (like scanning a book), you get the feeling of the whole process, and then you begin filling in the details. For each eye condition, symptom, or patient need, my approach is slightly different. The first step is to discover what your eye parts and measurements are trying to reveal.

In *What the Eye Reveals*, Denny Johnson claims that the iris—easily seen and studied with a magnifier or photographs—can be read like a map. Johnson's valuable contribution to the field of psychology is the ability to read the iris from the points of view of emotion and personality.

When you look at the remaining stump of a logged tree, you notice fine lines, concentric rings, and other markings that indicate the tree's age, growth patterns, and environmental influences. In the same way, the coloration and the spokelike patterns of the iris communicate familial tendencies and influences. The presence or absence of nurturing, creativity, commitment, anger, and fears can be determined from the crater-shaped (flower) or rock-shaped (jewel) markings on the iris. In addition, the degree of inward expression, accomplishment, purpose, peace and harmony, and capacity to be integrated between the different halves of our brain, and the link between our genetic inheritances, is also revealed in the iris.

At first, Johnson's form of analysis seemed too metaphysical for my scientifically trained mind. But a little voice inside me said, "Try it. Try it." I began conducting clinical trials using this Rayid method of iris interpretation (see the illustration on page 23). According to the Rayid method, three basic patterns are represented in the iris—emotional, kinesthetic, and mental. The fourth, the shaker (extremist), is a combination of two or more of the basic patterns. These patterns reflect the genealogical imprinting of the family tree transmitted to the offspring. Like a time bomb, these influences can be manifested as behavior at any time. In the Rayid method of iris interpretation, one compares the iris patterns of the left and right eyes. As I found in my clinical research, Johnson also found that the right eye represents the father's side of the family and the left eye represents the mother's side. If the right eye pattern tends to dominate, meaning more structural activity in certain places, it reveals left hemisphere dominance. In this case one could speculate that the father (right eye) may have had the greatest influence upon that patient's personality development. I would

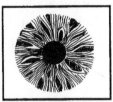

EMOTIONAL TYPE (Flower) has curved or rounded openings like petals. They are feeling oriented, **communicate primarily with images and learn auditorily.** Flexible, spontaneous and changeable, they flow easily in social situations, are animated, expressive, generate excitement, enjoy being on display. Living for the moment, their enthusiasm may be short-lived. They excel as artists, musicians, engineers. They need control so are attracted to MENTAL TYPES for long-term relationships.

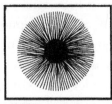

KINESTHETIC TYPE (Stream) has a uniform elongated fibre structure, revealing a tendency to believe that everything is their body. They like stability, are supportive and with true empathy create group cohesiveness and tend to serve and balance others. They **communicate by body posture (touch and movement)** and are naturals in athletics, dance, health care and public service. They learn auditorily, visually and by imitation. Because they need expansiveness, they attract EXTREMISTS (Shakers) in long-term relationships.

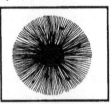

MENTAL TYPE (Jewel). Dot-like pigments on the iris indicate a thinking, intellectual person who tends to control self, situations and others. Precise **verbal communicators,** showing little emotion and using few gestures, they are often intense, deliberate, quietly driven people who enjoy pursuing goals. They combine well-defined views, attention to detail, commanding presence and excel as leaders, teachers, scientists. **They learn visually.** They attract EMOTIONAL TYPES for long-term relationships, who help them open, allow, feel, surrender and experience feeling rather than analysis.

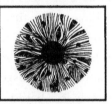

EXTREMIST TYPE (Shaker) has both dot-like pigments and rounded openings. They unify mental and emotional traits and communication modes. They are dynamic, progressive, unconventional in thought and action, at the forefront of change and challenge life with abandon and zeal, often drawing ridicule. Driven to achieve, yet ungrounded, they go through cycles of success and failure. Often devoted to cause and adventure, they excel as innovators, motivators, explorers. **They learn through touch and movement.** The Shaker really wants support and equilibrium, so is attracted to KINESTHETIC TYPES for long-term relationships.

A T T R A C T I O N

ATTRACTION

IRIS TYPES

correlate these observations to my own lens prescription measurements: was this person near- or farsighted, and was there astigmatism? Were the two eye measurements different? How did this correlate to the iris markings and the findings of hemispheric and parental dominance?

My clinical research took the Rayid method of interpretation a step further. I used the lens prescription findings and an in-depth case history, combined with the iris analysis, to explain how patients warped their vision perceptions in their mind. The iris gave me the background genealogical influences my patients had to deal with in order to survive in their family situations or general environment, which later molded the eye structure into a particular shape or degree of optical power. Conventional optometrists and ophthalmologists vehemently claim that near- and farsightedness and astigmatism are due to long or short eyeballs or misshapen corneas. In behavioral optometry, we see the eye deformity as being the end result of misperceptions from the brain and mind. My contribution to the Integrated Vision Therapy model is to study the role of family-tree influences, as shown in the iris, as a way of further exploring the developmental etiology of vision problems.

The degree of accuracy between the clinical correlations and the patients' genealogical influences astounded me. When I could not explain the perceptual adaptation of the lens prescription or the Harry versus Sally visual distortion, I looked at an enlarged photograph of the iris and discovered the following information.

My nearsighted patients tended to have dominant, controlling, mental/intellectual influences that seemed to stem from the mother's side of the family. This means that more jewel patterns are seen in nearsightedness dominant in the left eye, the mother's influence. The emotional or mental (intellectual) markings in the irises of nearsighted patients showed a preponderance of fear-based patterns, indicating that nearsightedness appears to be largely fear-based—fear of loss of love, fear of rejection or abuse, and fear of overbearing and severely disciplining parents.

If the patient is right-brain dominant, the left iris pattern reveals a stronger "will" influence from the mother's side. Such a patient could be acting out more left-brain behavior, such as analyzing, being overly verbal, and using excessive logic in order to seek balance. This may show up as controlling actions over men, depending on the Harry influences recorded on the iris.

Farsighted patients are dealing, by and large, with unresolved anger in the family tree. From a Rayid perspective, the anger can be carried down genetically in the form of unconscious tendencies toward angry behavior. The person will not necessarily demonstrate this anger, but still carries the potential to be angry. It is proposed that the likelihood of manifesting this anger grows stronger with each successive generation that carries this genetic information. (It is important to remember these influences are within the genealogy of four generations and sometimes do not show up in the immediate-parent relationship.)

Astigmatism can also be correlated with specific influences within the genetic makeup. Astigmatism means that the perception of clearness or blurring will be specific to a particular orientation of the axes of the eyeball. Typically the meridians or axes of the eyeballs are like orientations on a clock face, the right eye and left eye each having its own clock. There are two primary meridians, vertical (six o'clock) and horizontal (quarter before three), as well as oblique orientations (ten before four and ten after eight). Astigmatism occurs when the cornea assumes a steeper curvature in one of these orientations. By analyzing the refractive lens prescription of the eye, one can determine in which orientation the clearest or most blurry perceptions occur. Considering the iris structure relative to these corneal orientations, one can compare the genetic influence and the visual perceptual adaptations that have developed. If the orientation of the most blurred meridian is vertical, the lessons for the person to learn are patience, trust, and compromise. If the blurring is horizontal, then voicing one's inner truth through commitment is necessary. The oblique orientation of the blur deals with will and spiritual awakening, listening, and bringing forth hidden passions.

Studies of the vertical orientation of the body, considered by some to be the orientation of the human energy system (chakra system), indicate that the brain–eye pathway connects vision to the source of our soul in a creative or inspirational way. In order to be balanced, the various energy centers or chakras along the vertical axis need to be linked. This is another component of integration. Visual science recognizes two types of astigmatism, one in which the most blur occurs in the vertical orientation, and the other in which the blur occurs in the horizontal orientation. The most common astigmatism is the vertical blur, corresponding with nearsightedness. This is called with-the-rule astigmatism. The presence of astigmatism indicates that foundation perceptions are interfering with your ability to fully integrate your heart, ego, and soul. Ideally, optimal clarity will be found on both major axes. The amazing thing about astigmatism is that behavioral optometrists find the measurement of these eye distortions can fluctuate with changing thoughts and feelings. The degree to which measurements remain fixed indicates how ingrained are the the visual habits of the person, which of course relates to personality.

The more you are able to harness the power behind your eyes through flexible thinking, a dream, a vision, or heartfelt inspiration, the less intense is the measurement of the astigmatism.

Information from the iris is a key to subconscious variables that lurk in the dark cave of our visual perceptual consciousness. These controlling forces erode our power, and then we set up perceptual beliefs in an attempt to justify how we see ourselves. As youngsters we believe what our parents tell us about who we are, or who they think we are (good or bad, smart or stupid, and so forth). Our DNA molecules, as the genetic inheritance of our parents and grandparents, store one truth of who we might believe ourselves to be. In addition to this imprint, our brain cells hold a video-taped library of our perceived self molded by our various life experiences through our many senses. Our eyes are used to visually accumulate the majority of this videotape library to verify the accuracy of our perceived genetic self. This means that if our life experience of what we see does not match our genetically encoded belief of who we think we are, we mold our perceptions to survive our circumstances. This mental misperception later reveals itself biologically as measured vision problems in the eyes. Yet another aspect of self exists, and that is our essence, or light presence. Zukav calls this the soul. The soul may be the most important way of defining who we really are and what vision ultimately is about. The middle-to-late life quest to discover our true self requires that we let go of our limiting perceptions.

We now have the opportunity to decipher these visual adaptations and administer an Integrated Vision Therapy rehabilitation process that affects our whole consciousness.

Chapter 2

Opening the Door to the Brain

Storage of Life Experiences

Like a video camera, our brain tissue has the capacity to store the memories of our life experiences. Each moment of every event is meticulously filed in the videotape library of our minds. The recording process may begin earlier than our life itself.

The process of conception determines much of the future health and well-being of a baby. Your parents were responsible for the state of consciousness that was present, both for you and for them, at the time you were conceived. Ideally, that environment was rich with loving feelings. Because a human being's nervous system is sensitive to energy fluctuations, your father's sperm or your mother's egg may have been influenced by their respective thoughts, fears, and other factors present at the time of your conception.

A man and a woman on Earth once joined in sexual intercourse. When his sperm fertilized her egg, a new physical being was created. At the moment of conception, the chromosomes from "Dad" joined the chromosomes of "Mom," and two generations of family tree integrated to create "Junior." Perhaps the spirit of Junior chose to be on Earth and was able to manifest through this couple's union. The genetic foundation and blueprint of this new being, established in that instant, served as a way for Junior to verify the external "goings on" of his parents' lives. For example, Mom spoke in a specific tone under certain circumstances, and interacted with Dad and other family members in a particular way when under emotional distress. Junior checked the information on file in his genetic memory bank, comparing it with his notes on Mom's behavior. Any incongruence between these two caused Junior to develop physiological strategies of coping with his imbalanced perception. The same process was repeated with Dad. (Remember, this is just a story.)

Junior

Throughout the in utero experience, the little body of Junior was developing his senses of touch and hearing, and, by five months, he was reacting to light. Imagine the amniotic sac serving as an echo chamber, amplifying Junior's experiences of Mom and Dad. Junior's physical body and in utero experiences were being molded by the behavior of Mom and Dad and by life outside the womb. Then Junior was born. Depending on the circumstances, a whack on the behind in the hospital or a gentle transition into the loving arms of Mom at home, or any variation between these two, concluded Junior's prebirth experience. The prebirth and birth events were impregnated into his brain tissue, forming the basis for his perceptual development and the resultant molding of his body, including the structures of the eyes. This information would affect Junior throughout his entire life. "Junior" was named Shaun. For the next six years, Shaun continued the accelerated development of his perceptual life experience, which was constantly compared with his genetically encoded references. He went through the creeping, crawling, and walking phases, made the transition from breast milk to solid foods, and grew as Mom and Dad personally evolved. The family moved to a new home across the country. Dad and Mom held different jobs. His parents may have divorced, or perhaps they passed away. Shaun's number of taped experiences grew. Through speaking and moving his body Shaun was able to act out the incongruities between his genetic code and his life experiences through his senses. When his mind could not deal with what he saw, it would perceptually distort what he saw in order to let him survive, and over time this distortion would show up as a distortion in the eye, resulting in near- or farsightedness or astigmatism.

The previous story may seem surreal. Yet, physicians such as Thomas Verny and John Kelley, in *The Secret Life of the Unborn Child*, present convincing data about the richness of in utero experiences. Many people who are put under age-regression hypnosis can recall prebirth and birth experiences. The impact of all life experiences, including prebirth and birth experiences, that are at odds with the genetic blueprint may be held in memory in a special section of "the library" and then buried in the subconscious. The clarity of a present-moment experience is filtered through the past mismatches between what we "knew" genetically to be true and what our current experience reveals.

Anne

In Anne's case, the genetic memory was quite clear. She genetically knew her father was a loving and feeling man; however, when he acted in an inappropriately sexual way when she was a young teen, her perceptions were

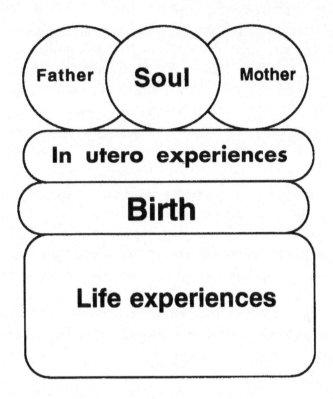

at odds with what she knew inside from a genetic and soul level. She did what she needed to do in order to survive, a strategy that included distorting her vision. One aspect of the coping strategy eventually revealed itself in astigmatism (physically, the cornea was shaped unequally and her perception in the right eye became warped and double). Without hearing Anne's story, I was able to see the genetic predisposition toward difficulties with sexuality from markings in specific locations on the iris. In assisting her clinically, we connected the relationship between her astigmatism and her sexual history. This alone produced enormous changes in her physical eyesight.

George

George was quite nearsighted at the time he discovered the power behind his eyes. As an adult, George had memories of his grandmother as a "hideously ugly" woman (she had a medical condition known as elephantiasis). George's mother, however, was a very attractive woman, and her beauty created a confusing duality for young George. During his first six years, he was never sure whether his beautiful mother or his fearful-looking grandmother would appear before his eyes. This visual duality caused him to be pulled off center and to not see in a straight, accurate way. George discovered that his severe nearsightedness was likely related to this severely

29

distorted duality in his perception of women, a reality so intense it affected George's capacity to have a deeply committed relationship with a woman. As George put it, he felt unable to find his truth in life and continue in a straight line because of this duality. George had already begun his vision improvement journey when he made these discoveries. His healing then went to a deeper level, and he was better able to understand the many causes of his severe eye problem.

My clinical interviews over the years compel me to believe that significant events in our lives are recorded in memory for later retrieval if we choose to raise our awareness. This gives us the opportunity to make new, healthy choices when we are ready. Reflect on any "videotapes" that are played out in your mind. Like George, many people who have cut off the memory of certain events are initially unable to access some of their videotape library. This blocking serves to short-circuit or disconnect the power within us. We stay in a restricted survival mode, coping with daily life instead of really living it.

The stories traditional peoples impart to their young carry an important message. The consciousness of youth is molded by tribal rituals, creating a cultural way of being that enables them to access their power within. Western children are being programmed by rock videos, television, shopping malls, and video games. These influences filter and distort the way they see life, creating the potential for further disruption of the "genetic" and "life" self. Imbalances affecting our internal capacity to be powerful cause us to behave like animals in the survival mode of fight-or-flight. This balance can be restored. Your power can be reactivated.

The Flowing of Our Energy

What mechanism has the ability to switch on our power and turn off the old videotapes that have been draining it? Power is derived from energy. Our primary fuels for stimulating our well-being are sunlight, nutritious food, plenty of rest, and a loving home environment. Other needs are our hobbies, recreation, career, and life purpose. How do you look for outside nurturing and love?

Healthy methods of maintaining harmonious balance—for instance, families taking the time to sit down and enjoy a meal together—seem to have been superseded by a materialistic, always busy way of life. Possessions, prestige, and "looking good" dominate our days. Culturally this distorted value system translates into "I am looking for love and nurturing outside of myself." Outside stimuli provide more gratification than our inner being.

Ultimately, the way we lead our lives affects our well-being and the flow of energy within us. We, as human beings, are becoming doers. In our survival mode, looking for outside stimulus, we grab fast food on the run and watch bad-news television before we go to sleep at night. Our power circuits become overloaded, which creates distress, according to stress researcher Hans Selye. He claims that *stress* in our lives is fine—*distress* is the killer. Selye's research has shown how animals' vital organs shrink when exposed to too much distress and imbalance.

To keep our inner power surging at manageable levels, we must create more balance in our lives. The life functions of the body are controlled by the autonomic nervous system, which is like a delicate seesaw. This aspect of the nervous system consists of many nerves that control vital organs and bodily functions. Balance is required between the sympathetic and parasympathetic branches of the nervous system. The activities of this nervous system are orchestrated by the hypothalamus, the master conductor of the body. Just as an orchestra conductor directs when each instrument enters and leaves the symphony and how loud it plays, the hypothalamus directs frequencies of light, received via the eyes, through the autonomic nervous system. This serves the purpose of keeping the bodily functions in balance.

When we are overstimulated (coffee, busy freeways, job deadlines), the sympathetic nervous system steps in and leads the way. Maintain this lifestyle for a while, and symptoms like chronic fatigue, headaches, flu, sinus congestion, indigestion, low energy, and short temper show up as warning signals. We are trained to respond to them by simply getting rid of the symptoms. Grab the antidote! Headache formulas, stomach antacids, and vitamins and minerals will "fix " the "problem," so we can continue, ad nauseam, to be busy doing instead of being. For some of us, the parasympathetic system takes over and we feel too tired upon waking to get out of bed. Our back hurts; our chest feels cramped. The body is clearly saying, "You need rest."

Mihaly Csikszentmihalyi, a psychologist from the University of Chicago, has devoted his career to the study of people who have developed the capacity to "flow with life," which he defines as learning to transcend time and literally *become* what we are doing. We can accomplish this and increase our energy by choosing activities we really enjoy. The juices of creativity are stimulated, physiologically speaking, and our distress levels drop. This form of being and living requires a commitment to be fully awake.

Tony

Tony arrived in Canada from Italy at age eighteen, with a suitcase in his hand and fifty dollars in his pocket. Wide-eyed and full of ambition, he set out to become financially independent and build a nest egg for his family. By the time he was forty, his workaholic personality (sympathetic-nervous-system dominant) was so revved that he devoted less and less time to his family and more time to creating "new business deals." His financial reservoir of millions of dollars, and his desire to make even more money, camouflaged the absence of a loving connection with his wife, who had long since left his bed. Like a shuttle train, Tony sped through life, ignoring the obvious breakdown in his life's balance, until the day his doctor diagnosed glaucoma in his right eye. (Glaucoma is increased pressure and lack of drainage of aqueous eye fluid.) The diagnosis implicated an internal buildup of pressure in his body and a loss of what Csikszentmihalyi calls "flow."

We could limit this metaphor to the eye. I prefer, however, to consider glaucoma's message as a life implication. Through the pressure to succeed in the financial world, with its accompanying upset of the physiological flow of energy in his body, Tony had created an unbalanced lifestyle for himself. At first, the message wasn't clear and loud enough, so Tony used drops in his eyes as he continued his busy life. Over time the doctors became perturbed, stating that his right eye was going blind. Finally, the body's message became clear to Tony and he decided to bring more balance into his life. The fact that his right eye was more affected than his left made him realize that his workaholic attitude needed to change. Tony needed to pay more attention to his Sally, left-eye side, and honor the part of himself that needed love and nurturing. He began by acknowledging that his marriage was not working. As he initiated changes in his life that reflected his true feelings and desires, he was able to reduce the medication for his glaucoma and take control of his own flow and power. While he continued to make money, he also developed a new, loving relationship with his children and with a new lady friend, balancing them with his continued aspirations.

Begin the journey of finding your balance and recharging your own power. Consider the following steps toward achieving awareness and making your life whole. You may wish to keep an ongoing vision diary as you integrate this learning. Use the pages in the book to record your realizations and feelings.

1. Reevaluate your life goals and priorities.
2. Adopt healthier eating patterns.
3. Set up a home life that is harmonious and flowing.
4. Identify previous incompletions.

5. If body symptoms exist, identify the significance of that communication. Initiate a self-healing course of action.

6. Lovingly take care of your physical body.

7. Ask yourself if you are really happy in your career or chosen work. If your career is your first and only choice, would you continue, even if you didn't earn money?

8. If you are in a marriage or a primary relationship, decide whether you are at least 80 percent fulfilled and empowered by the relationship. Do you find your mind wandering toward other potential partners? Does your relationship provide an outlet for spiritual unfoldment? Can you honestly state that your relationship provides a nurturing partnership?

9. Think about whether you devote time to recreational pursuits that are different from the type of work you do for money. For example, a computer programmer might paint for a hobby, while a landscaper or gardener may dabble in computers. A counselor or therapist might enjoy hiking mountain trails or windsurfing. These opposites activate balance of the nervous system and harmonize the brain hemispheres. Generally, you will feel refreshed after taking part in these complementary activities.

10. Try to live in an environment that supports your life purpose. So many of us choose a place to live because of the convenience of work and business opportunities, rather than choosing a place that nurtures our soul. Are you bothered by pollution, noise, electromagnetic interference, or traffic? Do you desire more space?

Healthier Eating Patterns

Do you prepare at least one meal, from scratch, per day? Have you considered that the vegetables and fruits you eat may have chemical residues? Consider beginning to purchase organic and unadulterated vegetables, fruits, grains, and legumes, even if it means spending more money. Do you consider your body important enough to feed it powerful and healthy foods?

Begin eating one freshly made salad and a variety of fresh vegetables each day. Lessen your intake of refined, processed foods, such as crackers, chips, and fast foods, and increase your consumption of complex carbohydrates, such as rice, barley, millet, and buckwheat.

The easiest way to reestablish balance in your nervous system is through a change of eating habits—getting back to the basics of ingesting fresh fruits, vegetables, grains, and legumes with varied seasonings, supplemented by animal protein (if you choose). Unlike dieting, eating for balance and power is a rejuvenating ritual, in which the kitchen is viewed as a creative studio. Food preparation is approached with love, focus, and purpose. Choose foods that will nurture and build your energy within. Your focus can be on nutritional sustenance and balance rather than on eating for gratification. For at least one meal per day, prepare a healthy spread (from scratch) using fresh foods with no additives or preservatives. Then, light a candle and dine. Enjoy this delightful form of self-nurturing alone or with friends.

Harmonious and Flowing Home Life

Look back to your childhood and your memories of home. Do you feel harmony during this reflection? Do you have negative emotional feelings about your home life as a child? If you could restage this period of your life, how would you design it differently? Now, consider your current home and the people with whom you live. Do you see any repetitions or similarities from your first home life? Look deeply for addictive or dysfunctional patterns and for where you are dependent. If your partner or other members of your household didn't return one day, would you feel helpless? The important observation is to identify where you might be giving away your power.

What factors do you need to consider in order to create more harmony and flow in your current situation? When did you last undertake a complete cleaning out of your possessions? If you haven't used an item in the past year, consider getting rid of it. Recycle it, give it to a friend, or sell it. This includes clothing, household appliances, and all personal effects that carry old energy and that may be unconsciously affecting your power. This old energy unconsciously keeps your perceptual mind focused in the past. The effect is similar to that of strong glasses, which force you to see life now as it was when the lenses were prescribed. In reality, this is your past way of viewing things. Staying in your past perceptions taints your current perceptions of life. Reclaiming the power behind your eyes is seeing the way things are now with fresh perceptions, unaffected by the past. Gifts, clothing, photographs, or belongings from previous relationships can keep you stuck in the past. When you unconsciously hang on to the past, your ability to encompass the present moment decreases. Your consciousness is bombarded by the past, and you may have difficulty being clear and powerful. Attachments of any kind, as to material things and thoughts, keep you from fully accessing your vast reservoir of creative power. Discover whether you have any attachments you would like to let go of. Your soul, your light, remains dim under the dominance of the part of you that seeks the security of the past.

Examine how you feel the next time your mind is occupied with many thoughts or nagging little worries. When you engage the thinking part of your mind, you probably will *see* less of what is happening in the world outside of your eyes. Incompletions get in the way of your natural ability to look at your daily life with clear, heartfelt love. Situations such as forgotten communications to friends or loved ones, broken agreements, unfinished projects, and suppressed dreams can affect your vision. Identify and write down any incompletions with family members, people with whom you work, and past relationships or jobs. What would you like to say to them in order to complete these cycles of your life? You will probably not need to take any action with the communication, either visualized or written, other than to complete the exercise for yourself. This sets in motion the necessary clearing within for you to once again activate your power of clear vision. For specific and intense situations you wish to clear, consider burning any material you have written, as a ritual or form of release.

Identifying Incompletions

Your body is constantly communicating to you. Every little ache and pain, release of mucus via a sneeze or cough, headache, blurry vision, and many other symptoms are your body's way of getting your attention. List the symptoms you have had during the past six months, including things such as falls or other accidents, bruises, headaches, nausea, upset stomach, hangovers, and so forth.

Paying Attention to Your Body

An exciting way to conduct this exercise is to keep a diary for a month, and write down everything that happens. When you read what you have written you will be amazed at the correlations between your internal process and the way your life manifests the exact learning necessary for you to wake up. It is as if your eye and body symptoms are the wake-up call to really seeing the truth as it presents itself now, not based on past, inaccurate perceptions.

One of the ways of generating power behind your eyes is to lovingly nurture your body and eyes. Make a list of the ways you would like to nurture yourself. Some of my patients' favorite ways are to have a full-body or foot massage; soak in a hot bath with mineral salts; take a sauna; go for a walk in nature; prepare a delicious meal; listen to classical music; have a facial, a manicure, or a hair cut; or spend time in the garden. These gentle activities are non–work-related and offer either physical conditioning or relaxation. Begin your self-nurturing now.

Another key to taking care of your body involves accessing the nervous system through body-mind relaxation techniques such as regulated breath-

Integrated Breathing

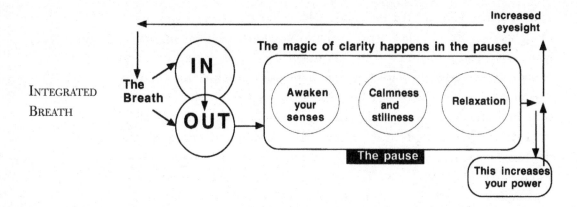

INTEGRATED
BREATH

ing. Of all the practical things you can implement as part of Integrated Vision Therapy, breathing is the most fundamental. Breathing is as basic to the program of vision therapy as the concrete foundation is to a house. One wonderful way to connect with your autonomic nervous system and to encourage and produce physiological balance is to begin a daily practice of integrated breathing and palming of your eyes.

Cover your closed eyes with your palms while you sit in front of an open window, breathing slowly and deeply and letting in the full spectrum of light. As you feel the warmth of your palms penetrating your eyes, feel yourself growing relaxed. Let all the strain and tension float away from your eyes and their muscles. Continue this for five to twenty breaths, or even longer. Then slowly remove your palms, opening your eyes and letting in the full spectrum of light.

Integrated breathing is fundamental to many of the exercises recommended throughout this book. Start by setting aside five minutes when you won't be interrupted. Find a comfortable place to sit or stand. Now when your eyes are closed, still and in their natural state of fluidity so you can focus on your breath without distraction, feel the oxygenated air entering your lungs through your nostrils. Explore the expansiveness of breathing. Practice extending the duration of the inhalation for increasingly longer periods of time. Notice the suspension at the end of the exhalation, and then inhale again. During this time of observation, pay attention to your chest cavity, particularly around your heart. Focus all your awareness on your heart and purposefully travel to the heart center.

Now, you will repeat the same process with your eyes open. At this point, use a flower, a candle, a familiar object, or a special photograph as a point of visual fixation. The new practice involves being able to keep the feeling of looking from the heart while in the presence of a visual distraction. You may notice that when your eyes are open there is a tendency to lose your awareness. Make sounds from the throat such as "AAAAH" for three breaths.

Do this exercise daily: Keep your eyes closed while breathing in an integrated fashion, listening to the sounds of life around you and within your own body. Then open your eyes and, while looking at an object with eyes fixed, continue the integrated breathing practice. You will soon discover that you can look at anything, even an emotionally charged "thing" such as a person, and feel love that is free of judgment, criticism, or the need to retreat or attack. This is a lovely way for you to personally balance your nervous system! This exercise provides healthy stimulation to your body and promotes your ability to relax.

Influences on the nervous system affect us physically, emotionally, and mentally. Mounting scientific evidence suggests that beyond and within the actual physical body, "fields" of flowing energy connect to our emotional, mental, and spiritual selves like a sophisticated telecommunication system. Our eyes, ears, and kinesthetic senses are the receiving devices for these energy fields. When we are healthy and balanced, these sensitive systems function at peak-performance levels—our vision is sharp, and we hear and feel beyond our "normal" abilities. We can literally feel vibrations from people and other living things around us.

We have all experienced momentary exceptional states where a higher capacity to see, hear, or feel is present: we know the telephone is going to ring; we see an event in a dream before it actually happens; our uncomfortable feelings about a person are later proved to be true. Imagine cultivating these aspects to the point where you can turn them on at will. Our conscious decisions dictate this capacity in our daily living. The way we use and abuse our senses determines the amount of reserve power available from our brain and mind.

For most of my patients, the notion that they can control their nervous system and brain is a totally new concept. Rather than being aware that we have a choice, we allow our daily lives to become robotic. We get up in the morning, go to work, come home, eat dinner, and fall into bed, repeating this habitual cycle ad infinitum, with the possible exception of a few weeks' vacation each year, at which time we attempt to relax. By learning to vary our activities and avoid negative, one-track states of being, we can reclaim the natural power behind our eyes. (I write more about this in chapter 8, "Renewing Your Vision.")

Mary and John

Mary and John had been married for fifteen years. She did all the cooking, slept on the left side of the bed, and put her toiletries in a specific spot in the bathroom. John always sat in the same chair at the dining-room table, always drove the family car when they traveled, and washed the dishes after every meal. This was their boring, rigid routine.

After consulting me, they introduced some variation into their daily lives. Just making small changes in the daily routine caused shifts in perception for both of them, similar to going away on holiday and seeing with new eyes on the return home or leaving a loved one behind for two weeks and experiencing fresh, new feelings for him or her on returning. Making such changes requires the brain to use different neural connections, encouraging a deeper interweaving of such aspects of the self as creativity, intuition, and intellect—which results in more power for seeing, feeling, and hearing.

Mary had been diagnosed as nearsighted. Her favorite pleasure was reading; she could devour a book in an evening. After coming home from her accounting job, which entailed spending six hours a day at a computer screen, Mary would sit down and read for another four hours. Most of her reading was done at night, under incandescent or halogen light sources. (Note: The color temperature of these light sources, in most cases, leads to an overstimulation of the sympathetic nervous system, preparing you for fight-or-flight, not relaxation and sleep.) By the time Mary wanted to go to sleep, her emotional and mental states were still hyperactive. When she finally did succumb to sleep, it was from physical exhaustion, not active choice.

Mary tended to be an intellectual person whose habitual state was to question things and compulsively analyze life. One of the first activities I suggested for her was to create periods of stillness: sitting quietly on the couch with a candle burning; taking a long, hot bath; or listening to music. Through these relaxation techniques, Mary's brain began to receive new communication signals. It said, "For this period of time it's okay to let go; it's okay to not think, analyze, and be logical." Mary began discovering other ways to *be*. Within a three-month period, her creativity in photography resurfaced and she entered a powerful phase of printing photographs she had intended to print years ago. They were, in fact, so good that her colleagues began purchasing them.

John loved television. A busy manager of a carpet warehouse, John relaxed in the evening by flipping on the TV and watching football, baseball, or movies. At the end of the evening he watched the news. John and Mary discussed world events before retiring, thus programming their brains with mostly sensationalized negative news prior to sleep. John's first assignment from me was to not watch television, read, or be busy *doing* for at least one hour before sleep. He varied the final activities in his day by preparing nutritious food for the next day, relaxing in the bath, writing in his journal (a newfound pleasure), or designing his dream home, a project that he could never get started before!

Mary and John now joined each other at least thirty minutes before bed, sitting quietly to discuss their day, talking from their hearts. Talking to clear the day's frustrations and incompletions before they went to sleep gave them the capacity to sleep more soundly, dream, and, through integration in the brain, begin the journey of developing their individual sense of wholeness. This, in turn, translated into clearer seeing, a greater capacity for listening, and living their lives with more compassion, feeling, and love.

Begin observing how your biological cycles are related to nature's cycles. Evening is the obvious time for resting the body and mind. When you are next tempted to turn on the lights and further stimulate your nervous system, experiment instead with stillness. Take a short, closed-eye break with gentle baroque-period music such as Vivaldi. Spend twenty minutes in that stillness. Then invest fifteen minutes in the creative state of pure being: write, draw, cook, or sing and move your body. In this way, your brain function is enhanced and other parts of your power are ignited. Mornings are for awakening the senses. As the sun rises and birds sing, activate the aliveness within you by stretching, moving your body, bathing, and preparing healthy food. Reading positive material in the morning can go a long way toward enriching your day.

Vision and Perception

Our primary sense is vision. The most obvious way we verify our perceptions is through the eyes. Michael Long, writing in *National Geographic*, exquisitely summarizes the mechanics of vision:

> *Sight begins when even a single photon from a distant star enters your eye and splashes down on one of a thousand raft-like cellular disks stacked in a rod photo receptor in the retina. On this tiny stage, molecules seem as big as boulders. The photon hurtles through a swirl of protein in the disk until it collides with a kinked sliver of a compound chemically akin to Vitamin A. In a quadrillionth-of-a-second twitch, the sliver straightens, much as you straighten your leg, precipitating a biochemical cascade throughout the photo receptor. The tiny footprint of the photon is amplified thousands of times to alter by mere millivolts the electrical signature of the photo receptor. Thus, light energy is changed to electrical energy, the hard currency of neural exchange. The signal now enters the cellular network of the retina for relay to the many higher processing centers in the brain.*

Scientists say one-third of the brain is designed to accommodate and integrate the signals coming from the eyes to be synthesized for vision. But what we ultimately *see* is constructed in the mind. Ninety percent of vision actually begins in the mind's videotape library, where our thoughts, feelings, and actions are stored. How and what we see begins with our self-image, those old perceptions stored in the imaginary videotape library in the brain. This is where genetic influences emerge and begin to have an influence over our perceptual experiences of life. During the first six years of life, we begin to construct a model of who we are, blending the genetic body with our life experiences. As we mature we may discover that we are housed in a body made up of our genetic influences, but we are not them. We are affected by our life experiences, storing those as part of our "life self," but we are broader than them too. The integration of these two selves serves as a model for our "real self," that is, how we think and feel about ourselves. The first sense of our real self contains strong influences of fear-based patterns and "rules for life" modeled for us by our parents. They also model their genetic and life incompletions, which reminds us of the aspects of our genetic self that we need to pay attention to. Ultimately, the real self is governed by our essence, our soul. I believe that the power behind your eyes is the power that helps you make this discovery, and then helps you to integrate your soul into the essential goodness of your genetics and life experience. From this place of recognition you realize that you are much more than who you think you are; you are able to say "I am of this body and of my life experience, but my essence is much larger than this physical expression." This is the ability to look with power from the inside. From this intentional point of view, you have the power to allow your real self to emerge and have every aspect of the life you desire.

Most of us see and experience life from two vantage points. We "think" life is one way and we intuitively "sense" it being another way. Our actual perceptions are activated by the interaction of the parts of our visual system: the eyes and the connecting pathways to and from the brain. Ideally, this system would allow you to perceive life as an integrated, unified state of being, but this state is usually quite rare in our busy lives. We would need to go to a deserted island or live in a cave for a few weeks before we experience anything similar to a whole-brain, multidimensional focused state: a state in which we are simultaneously able to access intellect and intuition. This is a particular way of doing while being, looking from your fovea while seeing much around you.

The scientific search for truth makes use of an oversimplified approach that reinforces the unilateral way of analytically and logically looking at things. Our educational system favors a similarly relentless exploration of knowledge through rational understanding—and it is no surprise that clinical findings reveal 90 percent of graduate students are nearsighted! Does academic study and the overindulgence in knowledge promote a nearsighted way of thinking? My clinical study shows students may lose some of their nearsightedness while on vacation, though it returns when they continue studying.

Transforming your relationship with yourself requires taking another look at who you think you are—your life choices, careers, partners, lovers, lifestyles, etc. Are your perceptions congruent with what your heart desires? Are you traveling down the path of your choice or a path long ago chosen for you through your genetic influence?

Joanie

Joanie was a successful, dynamic, and attractive actress entering a loving, live-in relationship at age thirty-one. Her presence was powerful and she exuded a "don't mess with me" attitude. She was affectionate and strong-willed, and she spoke her mind with an overtone of anger. Joanie initially consulted me because her right-eye vision was "lazy" and quite nearsighted, with astigmatism, while her left-eye perception was clear and mostly functional. When Joanie looked out through two eyes, she really saw only through her left. Joanie's sight was literally functioning on half-power, and she overcompensated for her right-eye perceptions. The eye printout was saying: "I'm not sure of my capacity to be clear and focused through my father's side of my genetic self, so I'll exaggerate those qualities to make me notice the situation."

Her assertive behavior that demanded she be heard and her clarity of speech were both exaggerated, in some cases to her advantage. Her voice-over career in commercial radio and TV was highly successful.

In other areas, Joanie felt incomplete. She felt unfulfilled creatively and was very defensive in the company of men. The limited perception of Joanie's right eye was affecting her orientation in life. This was confirmed genetically when we looked at the right-eye iris. A strong anger and clash-of-will pattern existed (see Rayid iris interpretation, chapter 1). In Joanie's situation, the "lazy" right-eye condition, her life choices, and the printout of the genetic coding on her right iris confirmed that the internal perceptions stored in her videotape library were affecting her being state in life.

Diana

Through unhealthy food and self-defeating inner talk, Diana had limited her progress to becoming an integrated, balanced woman. Her overweight body and narrow perceptions of life kept her very fearful. She was cross-eyed. Her eye condition reflected her inner state of being.

Using Integrated Vision Therapy, Diana began to reorganize her life to become more balanced. One of the activities for restoring this balance was to cover her TV screen with this written message: "I value my time enough to use other activities to evolve as a human being."

Chapter 3

Focusing your Mind

Only an awareness of your feelings can open your heart.
—Gary Zukav

Soul and Personality

What is the mind? Where is it located? How does the mind precisely direct vision? Can understanding the workings of the brain at a microscopic, cellular level help us know how vision ultimately takes place? Perhaps the psychology of perception can explain how light from a glorious sunset striking the retina is transformed into a dynamic visual experience by the observer. How do our thoughts, feelings, and beliefs affect the structure of our eyes? Is it possible that in every moment of living, we are sending subtle programming signals to the eyes—signals that affect the way life is viewed?

Many people think that the mind is located in the brain. However, this relegates our concept of the mind to only something physical. The mind is more than tissue or brain structure. Look at your mind as a total representation of all parts of your whole being. This appreciation will help you broaden the potential for promoting wellness of your eye structures and vision.

Your holistic mind includes your physical body. In your body lives your personality, a powerful aspect of "you" that is deeply influenced by your genealogy and parental conditioning. You may consider yourself to be merely your personality, the person who has a certain job, wears particular clothes, drives a particular car, or behaves in a specific manner. But tucked way somewhere else, perhaps within or around your body, is the immortal soul. And when the personality dominates, lacking integration of a deeper, spiritual connection to your soul, the imbalanced ego takes control to protect you.

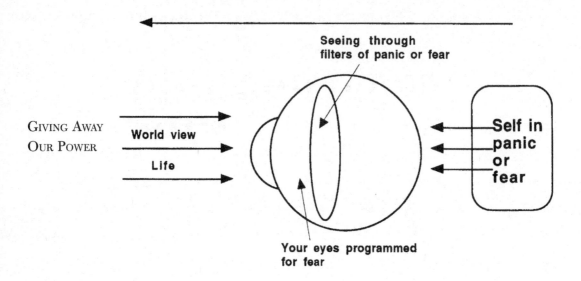

Your soul is the essence of your being, and persuasive evidence from near-death experiences and ancient Buddhist teachings supports the concept that the soul lives on even after the physical body ceases to function. Your connection to your soul serves as a way for you to link with love and compassion to all other souls, either visible in a physical body or unapparent. Gary Zukav says, "When you choose the energy of your Soul—you choose to create with intentions of love, forgiveness, humbleness, and clarity—you gain power. When you choose to learn through wisdom, you gain power." What behaviors do you notice in yourself that implicate a breakdown between your soul and personality? When you defy your soul in preference to the part of the mind known as the personality, you *see* through eyes of fear. Your vision is prejudiced with beliefs and judgment. You perceive your life as being outside of your immediate control. All power appears to be outside your reach. This way of looking sets in motion a perceptual sense of yourself as a victim. Your eyes respond as if this were the authentic way to behave, and the blood and nerve supplies respond accordingly. The next stage is for your eye and visual function to begin to break down, resulting in poor eyesight. I call this losing vision fitness.

Clinical observations support the theory that eye problems occur as a result of people's relegating the soul to being less important than earthly accomplishments. Refractive errors and eye diseases are external examples of a dominant survival-based personality.

Each eye anomaly appears to have its unique visual personality. Nearsighted individuals have an inward way of looking; they have more difficulty seeing the larger picture in a futuristic way. Their perceptions are more focused on the immediate present, and they focus on the present extremely well. I have often thought that I would employ only a nearsighted lawyer or accountant. I want these individuals to handle the detailed part of my life with precision and clarity. On the other hand, farsightedness is an outwardly focused visionary style, a far-reaching kind of vision. Farsighted people love to be philosophical, predictive, and speculative about future trends and changes. My marketing person must be farsighted.

While you increase your vision fitness at a physical level, it is imperative for you to begin reconciling your personality and your soul. Eye diseases indicate an exaggerated personality state, in which aspects of the soul of the person have been denied or the influence of the personality has been too strong.

Your personality state and the resulting perceptions may be traced back to your parents' or grandparents' lives. Blindness of perceptions in one generation, when unresolved, appear to be passed along and amplified in children and grandchildren. An example would be an inherent fear of loss of love. If the future parents live in this fear prior to the birth of their child, this emotional state will be transmitted at the time of conception. If the future parents continue to live in fear, then the evolving being, both in utero and throughout infancy, has the life experience of the same fear. The fear can be passed down energetically in the genes or vicariously via modeling by a parent.

If you ignore the truth of what your eyes reveal, your offspring may have an even more serious problem to resolve. For this reason alone, it is wise to look at your eyes as if they reveal a wonderful puzzle for you to solve. Whether you have children or not, when you deny your soul's perception, your own eyes will reveal this refusal to see in very physical terms.

The hypothesis that the new generation amplifies the incompletions, denials, and unconscious living habits of their parents and grandparents may help to explain the galloping increase in eye conditions and diseases in most cultures around the world.

An example of the way we allow the influence of personality to deny the soul, which could lead to a destruction of eye tissue, can be found in the way we interpret what we see happening to our planet. Consider the reduction of the ozone layer and the accompanying threat of skin and eye damage from the sun. A fear-based reaction to this very real problem may mean your health or your eyes actually will suffer from the ultraviolet rays.

Western allopathic medicine advises that we need to conceal our eyes and wear hats under all circumstances. Recently an Australian ophthalmologist suggested that all schoolchildren should be wearing sunglasses as protection from the vicious Southern Hemisphere sun. This paranoid attitude is a fear-based reaction coming from the personality; it is a denial of the soul, which entirely disregards the body's natural ability to use light for revitalization of tissue. This parallels the fact that nearsightedness is now measured in five- and six-year-olds, whereas twenty years ago it was unusual to find nearsightedness much before the age of twelve or fourteen.

Health is something that we have, not something that we get. Sunlight naturally stimulates well-being and counters the effects of harmful environmental influences upon the endocrine system. Research on Seasonal Affective Disorder (SAD) substantiates the benefits of using sunlight or full-spectrum light in treating depression: exposure to full-spectrum sunlight is necessary for robust vision and mental and physical well-being. Deprivation of full-spectrum light probably has more harmful effects upon health than does exposure to excess amounts of ultraviolet light. Absence of full-spectrum light promotes dental problems and hyperactive behavior in children.

A "soul-satisfying" way of looking at the problem of the diminishing ozone layer is to acknowledge the changes in the earth's atmosphere and still reap the benefits of the sun's rays. Try shorter exposure to full-spectrum sunlight in the early morning and late afternoon. In his book *Light: Medicine of the Future,* Jacob Liberman reports that by harnessing sunlight or natural light, you can restore the balance of the autonomic nervous system, which in turn harmonizes the control of the iris muscles of the eye. This equilibrium results in sharper focus of your mind and vision and will ensure that your soul and personality are acting in tandem—in a balanced relationship.

Arthur

Disease conditions of the eye are a means to observing the unfocused mind in action. Arthur, an educated man with a doctorate in philosophy, had been previously diagnosed as having an unusual disturbance of his right eye. Suddenly his vision in that eye went blurry. He had visited many prominent ophthalmologists, but no one was able to come up with a definitive diagnosis. Some doctors speculated that the loss of vision was due to an optic nerve disorder, but no specific therapies had been suggested. This affected his color vision.

Arthur had heard of the integrated approach to vision therapy, but he had never felt motivated to pursue a treatment. When the remaining vision in his right eye began to dim, he phoned me. It took going blind in his right eye to motivate him into action.

I spent almost an hour with Arthur during our first visit, integrating the variables of his life that could have contributed to the blinding of his vision. As his right eye was affected, I asked him to focus into his mind to find out how his relationship with his father influenced his choices as a man. Arthur was very perceptive, open, and intuitive. Predominantly using his left eye for so many years had trained him to tune into his soul perceptions. Arthur had actually given up his linear-oriented career path of teaching economics to begin a landscaping business and conduct personal-growth seminars. This is a clear example of how a particular perceptual consciousness can lead to lifestyle changes.

Arthur was not fulfilled, however. His soul and personality were still attempting to communicate an important message. Arthur needed to focus his mind's attention a little more. There was a missing piece.

The evidence surfaced during our consultation. He loved his new career helping people, yet he didn't seem to be able to make a financial success of the business. The clients he was attracting seemed to have money problems. While I patched Arthur's right eye and shined a yellow-green light into it, I had him begin to visualize the regeneration of the optic nerve tissue. I had him merge the healing power from his "soul mind" into his right eye.

Light has the capacity to stimulate emotions. Shining particular color frequencies of light into the eye brings emotions to the surface. This modality is a very useful adjunct in healing disease conditions.[1] With each integrated breath, Arthur tuned in to his assertiveness and strength from his father's side of the family. During the months that followed, his naked right-eye vision became more precise. This coincided with Arthur's working with more clients and reorganizing the financial aspect of his life. On a return visit to his ophthalmologist, he was able to pass a color vision test. Increased appreciation of color indicated a reactivation of his right-eye foveal vision. Arthur had harnessed the power behind his eyes to bring about clearer vision through his right eye and a greater integration of his two-eyed perception.

---

1. A branch of optometry known as syntonics uses specific frequencies of light for restoring visual imbalances of the autonomic nervous system that manifest in the eye as reduced side vision and upset vision measurements. The color combinations used are these:
   Green/Blue (turquoise), a parasympathetic stimulant, used to reduce inflammation
   Yellow/Green (lime), a slight sympathetic stimulant, used to activate release
   Yellow/Red (orange), a strong sympathetic stimulant, used to deeply activate release
   Blue/Violet (indigo), a deep parasympathetic stimulant, used to reduce pain
   Red/Violet (magenta), a parasympathetic stimulant, used to balance emotions

Paul

Arthur's brother Paul was less able to access his soul during our Integrated Vision Therapy. Arthur had encouraged his brother to see me. Paul had been born with congenital cataracts (clouding of the lenses of his eyes). The cataracts had been removed surgically when Paul was quite young.

In his teens, Paul had developed glaucoma, and he had used eye medication for many years. He also had a number of detachments of the retina. My first impression of Paul was of his enormous fear and mental-personality control during our first visit. I wasn't able to link with his essence or soul aspect.

The motivating force that brought Paul to see me was his fear of losing sight in his right eye. I carefully implied that the condition was based on something more than just physical trauma, yet Paul wanted only to know what vitamins to take for the condition. He couldn't yet see that his career as a computer programmer was hindering any form of rehabilitation of his eyes and vision. He said that working on the computer every day strained his eyes, but at this stage he was not ready to embrace the Integrated Vision Therapy concept. Once Arthur shared his success with using color, visualization, food modification, and the guided rethinking of his life, Paul returned to me for more assistance.

Paul was gathering information at the university library to try to understand how his glaucoma could be treated. He couldn't yet grasp the concept that his life choices, attitudes, and imbalance were contributing to his loss of vision. I welcomed him back, knowing that a part of his soul was ready to see in a balanced form. He told me he was feeling desperate about the ongoing loss of vision in his right eye. Paul was very afraid of going through a risky surgical procedure with no guarantees of success. He began using color therapy, and in spite of clear directions, he exceeded the recommended time of use. The pressure in his eye lowered and his field of vision began to expand. These results were most unusual from a conventional medical point of view. However, the success was short lived—Paul suddenly developed a further retinal detachment. His physician ordered laser surgery that day.

Paul's situation was complicated. He was not the usual Integrated Vision Therapy patient in that he did not yet seem ready to fully embrace his soul self. One could speculate that his long-standing history of eye difficulties, the color-light therapy, or some combination of both contributed to Paul's setback. I personally feel that the real variable in the downturn was that Paul's unconscious mind encouraged an overfocus of his dominant personality, resulting in his exceeding the prescribed time allotment in his color therapy treatments. Paul's idea of helping himself was that more color would be better for his eyes; his intellect dominated his application of the integrated vision therapy. He hadn't yet grasped that his healing forces would be activated by opening up to the power behind his eyes. I believe that when the person is ready to embrace his or her soul self, there is no longer any need to have additional physical reminders from the outside such as further eye-tissue damage. Perhaps Paul is still learning to trust his soul self. Until he discovers the power behind his eyes, which is not outside of himself in medication and surgery, Paul's eyes will probably continue giving him messages. Unlike Arthur, who approached his problem in a holistic way, Paul still looks outside of himself for the solution.

As an integrated vision therapist, I was challenged to accept Paul the way he was. I need to remember that when he is ready, he will return for the learning, or he will discover it somewhere else. This is the role of a facilitator: to let go of expectations and the need to try to coerce a patient into a certain way of thinking. As a patient, your task is to assert this desire to be a partner in your vision-care program with your conventional eye doctor. Getting to know your mind takes conscious observation. Begin watching your behavior. Either become your own visual detective or have friends or family members act as support in giving you constructive feedback.

You respond to the way you see life in two primary ways: (1) through your personality, you function from a place of fear, and (2) through your soul, you feel great compassion, forgiveness, and love in what you see. Integrating the two can be very easy; the challenge comes when you see things through the filtering system of your rigid personality. You may tend to respond in a reactive mode, and may then not be very receptive to receiving the requested feedback from your support person. Ask your support person to give you a signal as a gentle reminder when he or she perceives you acting from your personality self. Some of my patients ask their support person to use a particular sound, a hand signal, a touch over the heart area, or other such signals. Practice the integrated breathing exercises from chapter 2 to help you stay in a heart-connected way of looking at your behavior.

When you see from your personality, become aware of any feelings of fear. This ego-survival mind will have a repertoire of tricks to help keep you from facing your truth. The fact is that you wish to evolve as a soul. An opportunity, camouflaged as fear, has been presented. Your fear may override your soul's needs for a variety of reasons related to the past. The process calls for you to watch how you bring forth the reactions of righteousness, justification, rationality, negative self-talk, and other skillful ways of not facing your deepest self. The exercises and practices in this book are designed to stimulate your soul and to free you from the grip of your personality. As you exercise your mind and eyes in new ways, think of them as powerful muscles—not weak ones.

I See with Eye-C Charts

An eye chart may remind you of having your eyes tested. My Eye-C chart serves a different purpose. You use this chart to discover how your mind can bias your perception of the world. Through your eyes you will observe how your vision of the world can fluctuate. You will be putting yourself through different exercises and monitoring the ways that accessing various parts of your mind, your personality, and your soul can affect your eyesight. This biofeedback process will prove beneficial in understanding how you slip in and out of a balanced way of seeing the world.

If you have blurry eyesight at a distance, use the Far Eye-C chart. For close-vision blurriness, use the Near Eye-C chart.

For the Far Eye-C chart, position yourself at a four-, five-, or ten-foot distance from the chart, preferably without aid from any eyeglasses or contacts—that is, in your "naked," or natural, vision. For the Near Eye-C chart, stand the distance from the middle knuckle to the elbow of one arm. Ideally, you will be able to identify some of the letters in the middle of the chart. If not, move closer.

Notice whether you have any judgments about your seeing. This would definitely be your personality mind in action. Take note of your clearness of vision—that is, how many of the letters appear clear and at what distance. This will serve as the baseline level.

Begin the integrated breathing exercise. (Review this exercise in chapter 2, if necessary.) Open your eyes and observe the Eye-C chart to see whether there are fluctuations from the baseline level you noted when you first looked at the chart. Continue integrated breathing.

Does the clearness of the letters seem to fluctuate? Do the letters seem to stay about the same?

Remember a time in your life when you felt very happy. Notice whether this evokes a change in the way you perceive the letters. Now, recall an unhappy time and let the Eye-C chart communicate to you how your thoughts and feelings are affecting your perceptions. When you pay attention to what your eyes are saying, you can learn how to focus your mind to produce the vision you desire.

The Eye-C chart is a dynamic way for you to monitor the effectiveness

Near Eye-C Chart™

▲ vzuerpnrunduvenhndurpdhzenmyzkvzuerpnrunduvenhndurpdhzenmyzkmyzk ▲ (15)

frzezfvdxhpnfuqlmprnzfpzpnfrzezfvdxhpnfuqlm (20)

H P N V E Z F W H P N V E Z F W H P N V E Z F W H P N V E Z F V (30)

TH MARCOADZCNPQE KLSG J (45)

C B F R A O S Z M N D 2 (60)

L S F P O N Z 3 (7.5)

C D F U R 4 (10)

V Z F Y (12.5)

P R (17.5)

O (50)

▲   ▲

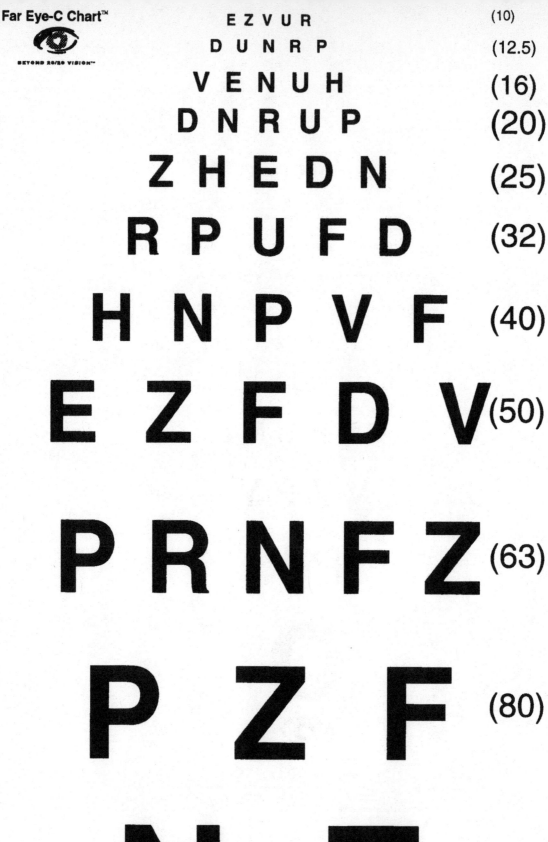

Far Eye-C Chart™

BEYOND 20/20 VISION™

Line	Size
E Z V U R	(10)
D U N R P	(12.5)
V E N U H	(16)
D N R U P	(20)
Z H E D N	(25)
R P U F D	(32)
H N P V F	(40)
E Z F D V	(50)
P R N F Z	(63)
P Z F	(80)
N Z	(100)

of your therapy. If your perception seems clearer through one eye, spend time covering the clearer-perceiving eye and repeat the process, looking through the other eye.

How clearly you see the Eye-C chart is a manifestation of your inner clarity—of how you use language, of what you see, of your view of your career, relationships, children, family—of everything in your life. As you traveled through adolescence to adulthood, you gained the intellectual maturity to deal with life's challenges. Was there a time in your formative years (or later) where you couldn't cope with what you saw? Perhaps that was when your inner clarity became blurry or when your two eyes stopped perceiving together. This unconscious adaptation was a protective measure I call self-sabotage. As you practiced this way of looking, your eyes began to respond as if that were the ideal way to see.

It would be great if I could say, "Just try this exercise or take this vitamin, and your eyes will get better." But if the process is to be successful, you must also take some responsibility for changing your vision, by exploring deeply your potential ways of seeing clearly.

Willingness to face your denials and deal with your reactive personality will lead to a state of what the Buddhists call mindfulness. Through your eyes, you will have a physical and physiological ability to stay focused on what you see. In this way, you observe your perceptions and behavior; then you are in a position to make energizing choices. Record weekly changes in your eyesight. Can you discover pleasant mental images that help you see the letters on the Eye-C charts more clearly?

Paula

When she first noticed her vision becoming blurry, Paula began integrated breathing and using the Far and Near Eye-C charts. She had never worn glasses and wanted to find out why her vision seemed more blurry when both eyes were open, compared with when she looked only through the left eye.

Paula had been experiencing discomfort above the right eye and had noticed that she tended to see images higher through the right eye than through the left. The baseline findings on the Far Eye-C chart confirmed her suspicion. The left-eye perception was significantly sharper, and when she attempted to look through both eyes, the right-eye blurriness interfered with her two-eyed vision. This is not an uncommon adaptation.

As I spoke with Paula, I learned that her Greek background was associated with very dominant male figures, particularly her uncles. The experience of being controlled by these authoritarian patriarchal men led Paula to partially shut down her capacity to feel safe with her male side. This meant that her perception of men influenced her ability to see clearly through her right eye. Her left eye dominated her vision of the world, with the right-eye perception hanging around in the background.

Looking at Paula, I couldn't tell she was seeing me in this way. The most apparent clue was her behavior toward me as a male. My experience of Paula was that she was very competent and efficient. If anything, she tended to dominate the conversation, maintain control, and turn her head sideways to lead from the left eye. I felt her to be controlling and overly strong from her masculine side. For the first level of Integrated Vision Therapy, I had Paula begin patching her right eye to stimulate her dominant-perceptual left eye. She needed to fully embrace the heart-connected feelings activated through the Sally side of her nature.

I had Paula look at the letters on the Far Eye-C chart and asked her to discover any feelings she had while practicing the integrated breathing. This was not very difficult for her because she was very bright, articulate, and could talk her way around her feelings. As she continued breathing, however, she was less able to hold back. The less I questioned her—reminding her of the presence of a strong male—the more she felt comfortable with the Integrated Vision Therapy process. Within a few minutes, Paula was able to hold the clarity of the letters. As she further focused her mind and integrated her new learning, she disclosed her choice of lesbian relationships. We discussed the likelihood of her perceptual adaptations being linked to these preferences.[2] Our conversation began to feel more connected.

As she began to feel more, Paula was able to bring heart and love into her still-powerful right-eyed perceptions and way of being. She deepened the practice of speaking about her feelings while looking at the Eye-C charts by switching the patch to the left eye.

It would be interesting to note the changes her relationship moved through once Paula integrated her vision more deeply and focused her mind in this balanced way. I have seen cases in which a client, secretive about her choice of a lesbian relationship, moved into full acceptance of this choice as her vision integrated. In one case, a client moved in with her female partner and got married. They fought the discrimination of the local gov-

---

2. In my case studies, women who choose lesbian relationships demonstrate a pattern of visual findings that deserve further clinical investigation. I encourage other clinicians to observe and research connections between perceptual distortions and sexual inclinations.

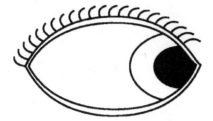 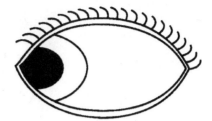

EYE
CROSSING

ernment, which did not permit two people of the same sex to join in marriage. More research is needed in this area; there are many questions to consider. In Paula's case, would more connective loving vision from her soul lead her to different choices?

Cross Your Eyes—They Won't Get Stuck!

As children we were taught that crossing our eyes is dangerous and can lead to maladies, that crossing our eyes will make them stay that way. For more than fifty years the practice of eye crossing has been taught as a vision-therapy technique. If you have any fear that your eyes will get stuck, please know that this is a very safe procedure. There are muscles for eye crossing and uncrossing. Even young children and adults who have crossed eyes are taught how to cross their eyes as a way to learn how to uncross them.

I heard a very funny story from a patient, Sam, who was warned that a certain part of his anatomy would fall off if he crossed his eyes. He could read for only twenty minutes before his focus wandered. He became irritable with this situation, which led to a loss of self-esteem. It turned out that crossing his eyes was exactly the therapy Sam needed. The simple practice of crossing his eyes helped him enormously. Sam was able to read and maintain comprehension, not fall asleep while driving or doing desk work, and stay sequentially focused on a project and finish it. He developed more discipline in his life and began to accomplish things that he had only dreamed about. Let me take you through some of the practical exercises Sam learned; they may help you, too.

Nose Crossing

Light a candle that has a medium-sized burning wick. (When the candle is lit, the flame should be clearly visible.) Sit two to three feet from the candle, which should be positioned below eye level. This will be easier for you to aim your eyes and not become fatigued.

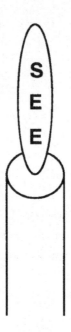

Begin integrated breathing to bring about a relaxed, heart-felt state. Close your eyes and feel all the tension leaving your eyes, neck, shoulders, chest, stomach, hips, and the other parts of your body. While your eyes are closed, listen to the sounds around you. Imagine you are lying in a warm bath and you feel very comfortable and calm. Let go of your daily tasks and imagine a peaceful life without any worries. Maintain this image for about twenty breaths. See the flame projected onto your closed eyelids. Focus on the flame, then move your attention around the edges of the flame. Keep breathing and appreciate the color of the flame.

Open your eyes slowly and look directly at the candle. As your eyes join the candle, breathe. Notice objects around the candle and in the room as you look into the flame. This is looking while feeling. Also, blink while breathing. After twenty breaths, cross your eyes and focus on your nose as you attempt to see both sides of it at once.

If you are unable to see both sides, patch the eye that corresponds to the side you can see. Train your other eye to turn inward by again looking at the tip of your nose. Repeat this part of the exercise until you are able to see both sides of your nose. Notice the candle flame while you practice the "nose crossing." You should see two candles. If there aren't two, blink for two full breaths to stimulate both eyes into seeing two candles. If you are unable to see two candles or both sides of your nose, abandon this vision game, and continue patching one eye to develop greater awareness through the open eye.

Remember what each eye represents in terms of perceptual consciousness—right, father perceptions; left, mother perceptions. Bring that awareness in through your open eye. Soon you will see two candles and two sides of your nose. Nose crossing teaches you to be more centered. This vision game is useful if you are farsighted. It is the beginning of fusing the perceptual channels of the left and right eyes. This is the initial step for merging your soul and personality consciousness.

While looking at the candle, see whether you can become aware of both sides of your nose, one side at a time. Breathe and blink to have this experience. If you have difficulty, alternate your blinks, identifying where each side of your nose is in space. Raise your chin to see the sides of your nose more clearly.

Nose and Eye Uncrossing

Choose an object of interest beyond the candle such as a flower, a painting, a photograph, a light, a window, or a personal object, and look at it with both your eyes open and uncrossed. Position the candle between your eyes and the object you are looking at. Become aware of the presence of two candles.

By looking past the candle, you are now creating a double perception of the candle. This mode of looking is asking you to let go, to uncross your perceptions, to diverge and be open. Observe the way that varying your attention can create separation of the two candle flames. Uncross until you

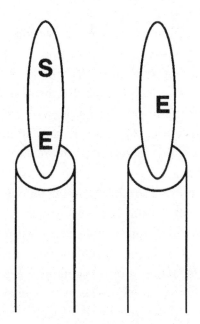

have maximum separation of the candles. Then move the candle toward you, observing how the two images of the candle appear to come closer. This "eye uncrossing" is particularly helpful if you are nearsighted and have astigmatism. Play this vision game when you wish to take a break from reading or working on the computer, or when your eyes feel tired or get blurry. Then use the two-candle illustration (on page 57) and create a third candle in the middle by crossing and uncrossing your eyes. Align the SEE in a straight vertical line.

Eye Crossing

Now cross your eyes as if you were looking toward the center of your eyebrows. In this way, you will be able to notice the two candles beyond where you are looking. If you find this difficult, first put your thumb or a finger in front of your eyes to remind you where to look. Once you have mastered eye crossing without a finger, stand up and walk around, seeing everything double. Breathe and enjoy this new perception. Observe how your balance is affected by seeing everything in twos. Can you let your attention move from one image to the other?

Multi-dimensional Vision

When your perceptions from each eye are close to being equally clear, you can begin the journey toward multidimensional vision. Position your two thumbs in front of your eyes. By crossing or uncrossing your eyes, you will begin to see either four or three thumbs; the goal is to fuse the four into three.

Computer-generated targets like the one on page 59 have created many new possibilities for fusion games and for developing a multidimensional way of being. When you cross or uncross your eyes so that the two black dots in the illustration become three, let your attention move down into the center of the page. Suddenly a three-dimensional form will emerge from or sink into the page. Stay with the image, and the depth will continue. Breathe, and move your attention gradually around the page. Practice moving from the crossed to the uncrossed position, each time noticing the image in the picture change.

Attempt to do this exercise while standing on one foot, walking around, and even trying to spell difficult words backward.

How long can you hold your visual space? If you have a weaker pair of eyeglasses, experiment with wearing them while doing this vision game. This is the way to restructure your perceptions. Focusing your mind while you stimulate your vision through your eyes teaches you how to be with

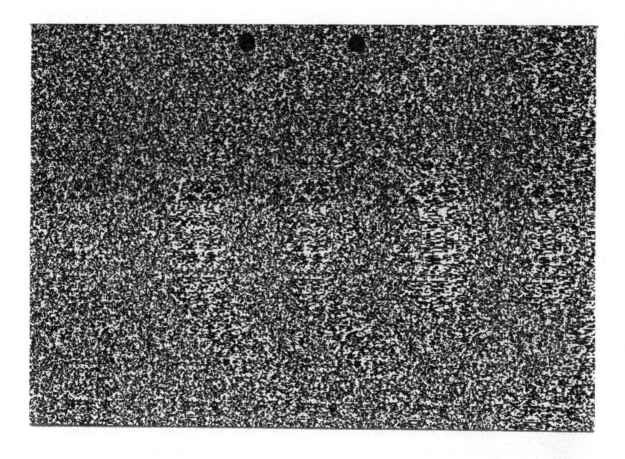

yourself and allows your soul to emerge. Review the activities in chapter 2 now that you have begun focusing your mind more clearly. Pay particular attention to activities that you resist. Gently move into the resistance. This is where the real healing begins.

Your soul *sees* only with love. Breathe and feel your heart open to this clear vision. Goodness emerges from a clear heart. Focused vision from your mind brings love and light into your life.

Chapter 4

What Do You Want?

Awareness and Healing

One of the initial statements I have my patients consider is: "With regard to my eyes and vision, what I want is . . ." They are then asked to write five different endings to that statement. The way you approach this question reveals a lot about your self-image and your view of life. Try the exercise for yourself.

Both the eyes *and* vision are mentioned in the statement. If you haven't yet made the leap to the concept that vision is 90 percent in the mind, please do so now. Close your eyes, and while feeling your breath travel below your throat, breathe into your heart. Keep your mind very still, and deepen your appreciation that only 10 percent of vision occurs through the eyes and that your mind holds the mystery of the other 90 percent. Now, look again at your five responses to the statement.

Many of my patients at first limit their vision by considering only what is happening in their eyes. At first, their responses might include:

- to have better eyesight without my eyeglasses
- to not need glasses for reading
- to fix my glaucoma
- to throw away my contacts and eyeglasses
- to remember more content and read more efficiently
- to get rid of my floaters (the spots or wisplike things that move in your line of vision)
- for my cataract(s) to disappear

In Western culture, we are programmed to look only for end results. But integrated vision demands seeing deeply and passionately into the *process* of how we see, exploring the mechanism of our unique mind-eye relationship. We see with our minds through intellect, a logical process of analysis and understanding that I call the personality, and with intuition, a divine inner knowing—the soul. You are learning how to integrate the two processes to achieve balanced foveal and retinal vision. The question, "Why bother? We're going to die anyway," may even arise. The personality part of us probably just wants to survive—that is your ego. But the joy and excitement of being alive and having access to the power behind your eyes has to do with *quality* rather than *quantity*. Can we live our lives today, experiencing the quality of every moment? One of my patients put it this way:

> *I wake up in the morning and there's a stillness around me, like in a desert. Not a sound. I feel so expansive, like my senses can reach out for miles. I feel fully present with myself and am empty of worry or thoughts. A pleasurable sensation of ecstasy moves over me like a warm hand. Each moment is frozen in slow motion and I am free.*

This ecstasy state contributes to the regeneration of our bodies. Second by second, each cell that makes up our physical mass is being regenerated, and our senses—vision, hearing, and feeling—are being finely tuned. The sound of a racing car's engine is music to the mechanic. The eyes of a photographer or artist are accurately synchronized with the mind-state to *see* the final rendition of his vision: the completed work. The musician hears at frequencies that the average ear misses and must be trained to perceive. The Olympic athlete mobilizes muscle groups in his body that integrate circuitry in the brain beyond that of the average individual. This capacity, beyond the normal, harnesses and directs the power within. A deeper commitment to being connected with ourselves gives us access to that power and fosters daily healing and regeneration.

As you integrate the personality and the soul parts of yourself, you become connected to the continuum of life that is represented by nature. Your perceptions reveal to you how everything is linked. An action of ten years ago can profoundly affect this moment. The natural healing process of your body constantly talks to you through the symptomatology of the aches, pains, and life stories revealed through disease. The story revealed through your body or eye problem is talking to you. It is telling you that you are out of balance. You need to integrate more. This is the truth. We can blindly choose to ignore the truth, until, one day, "all hell breaks loose," and we speed up the inevitable approach to death. The alternative is choosing to stop the disease now.

A patient who had completed a personal-growth training in order to be more accountable in her life told me this story: She was driving down a major freeway where the speed limit was fifty-five miles per hour. She felt excited thinking about the wonderful possibilities ahead of her in her life. Checking her rearview mirror, she saw the flashing red and blue lights of a police car. She glanced down at her speedometer. The needle was pointing to seventy-five. She pulled her car over to the side and rolled the window down, waiting for the officer to come over. A strange feeling moved through her body, quite unlike her past experiences of pondering how she could coerce the cop into believing her excuse. She felt a vibrational movement, a warm blast of heat stimulating parts of her physical body into being totally present and awake. She felt this warmth for a moment before the officer appeared, asking for her driver's license.

What followed was a spontaneous, unplanned response that was to change this woman's life forever. She turned her head and said, "Officer, I realize I was going too fast. I'm grateful you were there to remind me. I could have killed somebody." This visibly caught the highway policeman off guard and he asked the woman to accompany him to the highway patrol office. He wanted to introduce her to his superior because, in his career, he had never been thanked or acknowledged for his job.

He didn't issue her a ticket, and this woman's life was strangely altered. She now realizes that every action or choice she makes affects every aspect of her own life and of those around her. She is not interested in focusing on the part of life that is called disease. That's like looking at a half-full glass of water and saying it's half empty. Her new power is to acknowledge the living time available in her life which, from now on, will be high-quality awareness, moment-to-moment nurturing of the power within her.

This connection to the self heightens our senses, and the quality of our daily experience is enriched. This place of healing allows us to identify the warning signals that alert us to mental and physical breakdowns before they happen. It's like having our own police officer with us to flash the lights when we're speeding through life too quickly.

Healing is being awake and seizing every crisis as an opportunity to identify the breakdowns and see them as specific and helpful messages. Healing involves the regeneration of all those parts of ourselves that want to have a say in how we live: the artist, the parent, the entrepreneur, the lover, the child, the businessperson, the student, the cook, the athlete. Each aspect of ourselves contributes to the whole person we are or know we can be. To be clear and powerful we must maximize our health in each moment, embracing every moment with all the energy and focus we have. Every action counts.

As a young boy, I found school very challenging. With my double vision, nonreading habits, and farsighted perceptions, I would be physically sitting in class, but my mind was already bodysurfing in the ocean. I recall the excitement of anticipating the upcoming summer holidays. I could project weeks into the future. I imagined myself going to parties, eating, and hanging out with my friends. This mind-set of escaping the present moment reinforced a genetic, farsighted, family pattern of *looking*.

Over the years, this habit kept me from fully embracing the moment I was in. When the holidays actually began, I was in heaven. Yet my mind was already focused on the fear of how these good times would end. Even though my holidays lasted for two months, as I was returning home from college or driving with my family to our vacation cabin, my mind would be accessing the place called "worry." "When I return back along this route in two weeks or two months, how much work will be waiting for me at university next semester?" This way of *seeing* life was reinforced by my poor academic achievement and my father's criticism of my scholastic abilities.

The lesson I am learning is to pay attention to every moment of my daily process. I remember a time in Amsterdam when I was interested in seeing a movie but couldn't find the cinema. Eventually, in the dark foyer of a hotel, I located a newspaper to find the starting time of the movie. The small print was too much out of focus for me to clearly read. I noticed my impatience, stopped, took a deep breath, blinked, and the print popped into focus.

You too can become aware of your journey and your vision. Enjoy the day-to-day content of life; embrace the total experience. Begin identifying the habits of escape that keep you from fully enjoying yourself in the moment. Become aware of what you want right now.

Here are some questions to ask yourself immediately upon waking each day:

- What is the first thought that runs through your mind?
- What dreams do you recall?
- How long do you remain in bed?
- What does "today" feel like for you in that moment of awakening?
- Is your mind racing to the "doing" part of your life? Can you slow down? Can you break your habitual patterns?
- What new approach can you put into use that will express another part of your inner power?

- Are you focused on thinking? feeling your body? responding to someone else's needs? Do others depend on you, or vice versa?

- What new activity, exercise, or process could you initiate while still lying in bed? Perhaps you can do something different this morning: go for a walk; delegate a regular task to another person; stretch your muscles; read an inspirational book; light a candle.

- Are your plans for the day consistent with your long-term purpose? Take a few breaths. Instead of grabbing for your glasses, be in your naked vision. Put on a patch. Palm or shift your eyes from one point to another.

Explore these questions and write down your thoughts. I find that spending a solid ten minutes writing about my feelings every morning gives me plenty to reflect on throughout the day.

The act of writing is a marvelous way to ground and become clear in your mind. Take one aspect of your life and write your thoughts about it. Bring your powerful clarity through your hands onto paper. Complete some letters you wish to write, or jot down insights you wish to bring out into the world. Your written page serves as the beginning step to actualize your vision in the physical universe. When your eyes receive clear communication from your mind, they begin to see with balance and sharpness. You will notice momentary flashes of clarity while reading your Eye-C chart. With time, this clarity will linger for longer and longer periods of time. Soon your life will mirror this power and clarity.

Determine the hours when you, with your unique physiology and biochemistry, are the most productive, creative, supportive—or in need of support. Our bodies respond differently to the cycles of day (light) and night (dark), and we can maximize our power by getting to know our true preferences, which are sometimes *not* aligned with our present patterns. As much as we have been programmed to believe that routine is important, breaking inflexible habits that restrict our vision sometimes requires modifying our daily routine and controlling our behavior. To feel more alive and fully in your power, begin altering your perceptions of who you are. Here are a few relevant questions to ask yourself, and suggestions for action.

- What special things will increase your well-being in the moment? Perhaps you can give yourself a foot rub, run a hot bath for yourself, or serve yourself breakfast.

- Do you wake up at the same time each day? Vary the times. Experiment with waking up one hour earlier or one hour later. Occasionally get up in time to watch the sunrise.

- Do you feel as though you need an external stimulant such as coffee, a hot or cold shower, or a five-mile jog to get you going for the day? If you normally wish to go out and run five miles, spend that time listening to quiet music and stretching your body.

- If you are usually quiet, with low energy, do something that ignites your fire. If you tend to be slow and not move much, go out and do some power-walking.

- Do you have strong beliefs that you are a morning, midday, or afternoon sort of person? If so, then switch the times you do your most important activities for the day.

- Do you grab for your eyeglasses or contacts in the morning? Do you notice that your eyesight is more focused or less focused in the mornings? If you wear eyeglasses or contacts, leave them off for a few minutes or hours longer. Experiment with how you feel when negotiating known areas in your home without using artificial lenses. Enjoy the feeling of slowing down your pace, and enjoy the need to feel your body more.

- Have you an established eating pattern or other routines within the first few hours of the day? If you usually skip breakfast, make breakfast your main meal of the day for a while.

- Do you tend to talk a lot or to be quiet? Change your pattern.

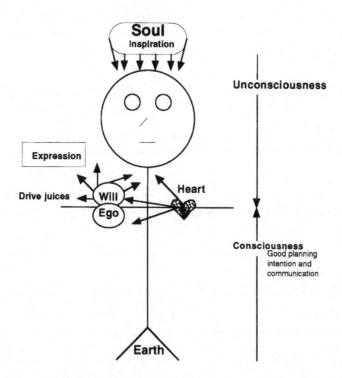

I have been suggesting that you begin consciously watching your habitual patterns. Are they performed by choice, or are you unconsciously playing out some influence from your mind that limits your potential as a human being? Your observations will permit you to see all the pieces of the puzzle of your visually related behavior. As you implement this process, remember that psychologists generally believe it takes three weeks to three months to learn or discard a habit.

After at least three weeks, then, you will be ready to again write your responses to the statement "With regard to my eyes and vision, what I want is . . . ." This time, please consider a second statement: "The way I'm likely to sabotage what I want is . . . ." By getting in touch with your unconscious habit patterns, you will become aware of the ways you hold yourself back and give your power away with negative thoughts, limiting beliefs, procrastination, fear, and laziness.

Playing with Resistance

In your journey so far you have entered the doorway to your vision—your mind—and have looked at your unconscious habits. Becoming aware means waking up to your past restrictive vision.

Your subconscious is like a lush, fertile oasis in the desert of your mind. It is your divine intelligence, storing treasures and riches; it is your *knowing*. The desert of your mind is the watchful guard protecting you from the perils of living. Those limiting beliefs include "It is dangerous out there," "Others are going to take it away from me," "The name of the game is survival."

While growing up, most of us had to adopt a "survival mode" of processing life. We came into life with the power of the oasis, but for many, this creativity had to be sacrificed to (or protected by) the rational ego—the survival mind.

Knowing what you truly want necessitates facing both the desert and the oasis. The desert can be thought of as foveal doing, while the oasis is the retinal being. In this process, you will explore your resistance to unlimited knowing and to the powerful action of integrating the power behind your eyes. Through becoming aware of what you resist, your dreams, intentions, and vision become clear.

The three forms of resistance can be categorized in metaphor as papier-mâché, plywood, and a brick wall. As we go through life, our resistance appears in variations of these three forms. The stalwart, traditional approach of using eyeglasses, contacts, medications, and surgery is a brick wall—the most resistant, rigid approach. If something is wrong with your eyes and vision, a doctor corrects it by covering or fixing the problem. Behavioral vision therapists who incorporate integrated therapies are less resistant—like plywood. The least confrontational, the papier-mâché, is most easily dealt with. The brick wall is the most challenging.

Annie was 65, happily divorced, and living in a house she had occupied for twenty years. She consulted me because she was developing cataracts in both eyes, and her ability to continue driving was being threatened. She wondered if there was anything I could do to help her.

Annie

I explained that the word *cataracts* literally means "like a waterfall," and asked her what experience from the past might be clouding her present and future vision. I noticed her fold her arms tightly across her chest, a physical position of resistance. With some covert hostility, she asked me what I meant. I said, "Cataracts can mean there is something in your past perception of life that is obscuring your vision today."

As Annie pondered my statement, I reviewed a summary of the food she had eaten in the previous two days. Scientific evidence is demonstrating that the consumption of dairy products disrupts the metabolism of the lens of the eye (where the cataract develops) in people who are lactose intolerant. Also, the presence of free radicals, vitamin scavengers, have become a problem for our eyes. The extra pollutants in our air, food and water have increased the need for antioxidants such as selenium, zinc, super oxide dismutase, chromium, and vitamin A. If the number of free radicals in the body and eyes exceeds the presence of antioxidants, the eye is predisposed to developing cataracts.

As I watched Annie, I could feel her internal fight between being in the desert and being in the oasis. One part of her being, the all-knowing oasis, was saying, "Yes, yes. I know what you're talking about." The desert-guard, the rational personality and ego-mind, was saying, "Just tell me what I need to eat in order to make my cataracts go away—if that's even possible. None of this psychological mumbo jumbo please."

Integrated Vision Therapy is a mingling of traditional vision therapy concepts and spiritual practices such as ritual dance, sound, and movement, and the use of color from the ancient civilizations of Egypt, India, Tibet, and Africa. We don't necessarily desire to give up the protection of the desert around us. It lets us focus on the unlimited resources of the oasis. In Annie's case, she did just that. She looked back in time and explored the twenty years of personal baggage that was preventing her from reaching her present life goals.

"I want improved vision, to continue to drive my car, and to lead a productive life," she kept saying. We devised a plan to bring this clear intention into reality.

Annie's assignment was to clear out the clutter that had accumulated in her home and was preventing her from *seeing* the space. The collection of boxes, papers, and artifacts from her previous marriage was no longer serving her. Once Annie saw how these obstructions were connected to her cataracts, her resistance went from brick wall to papier-mâché. I call this process "breakthrough."

I have noticed with other patients that breakthrough can be preceded by other processes. One is "breakdown." For instance, as I began to see the light in my own life and to be clearer about my own direction, things seemed to get even worse for a while. Not long after my own divorce, I was happy to be free and yet very emotionally volatile. In a period of three weeks, I got stopped three times by the police for speeding. Breakdown.

Following this phase comes what I've termed "breakopen," a step toward breakthrough. In breakopen, you can feel and see the greenery of the oasis around you. Your vision becomes clearer. This is the integration of the soul and the personality. In Annie's case, we used several approaches to deal with the cataracts.

First, Annie committed herself to a six-week process of cleaning her house, eating differently, using food supplements, and listening to a visualization audiotape I designed specifically for her, to help reprogram the metabolism of the cells in the lenses of her eyes.

Once a day she prepared a meal that consisted of miso (soybean paste) soup with sea vegetables (hijiki and arame), combined with a variety of vegetables. Fresh fruits and organic vegetables, grains (rice and millet), and legumes (mung, aduki, and black beans) became her mainstay foods for twenty-one days. The food was supplemented with a glandular-based multivitamin and mineral supplement, antioxidant enzymes from wheat grass, and "Eye Bright" eyewash, which includes eyebright, bayberry bark, goldenseal, raspberry, and a small amount of cayenne pepper.

Each day, Annie listened to the audiotape I had made for her, which suggested, through imaging, that her cataract material was dissolving. The image was that she was going inside her eye as a miniaturized person, carrying a doctor's bag full of useful remedies, homeopathic preparations, and color and laser-light machines that she could apply directly to the lens of her eyes. In this visualization, Annie became her own healer, using complementary approaches. (A branch of the National Institutes of Health is funding research to investigate these types of alternative healing practices.)

Annie also began to systematically clear out of her house anything she hadn't used in the past twelve months. I suggested she give everything away or sell the items at a garage sale. As the weeks went by, Annie saw minor changes in her vision, and by the end of the third week, she felt her long-lost self-confidence returning. She visited her ophthalmologist, who was not informed about the self-healing she had been conducting. With a puzzled look he scratched his head and told her the cataract material had dissolved by as much as 30 percent. Her eyesight had improved enough for her to realize her dream of continuing to drive.

I spoke with Annie months later. She was still driving and living in the oasis, free of resistance. She knew what she wanted. She went for it, facing the resistance and breaking through the barriers of her personality. This awareness returned her power behind her eyes. She was able to transform her relationship with an eye condition previously considered hopeless. The benefits far exceeded her original goal.

This Is It

The controlling influences passed down through our family tree and from our early life experiences can keep us from seeing fully today, and from clear vision. One of my earliest experiences with personal growth and transformation was the statement: "This is it—your life is not a dress rehearsal."

As a farsighted person, I mused on my habit of always planning for the future and treating the present as only a practice session. On my fortieth birthday, I adopted a "this is it" form of living. I wanted to be fully present in as many moments of the *now* as possible. I learned and then began teaching the principles of personal accountability. These were brought home to me by my interaction with a particular patient in the 1980s.

I met Linda in 1982, when she consulted me to deal with her nearsightedness and astigmatism using Integrated Vision Therapy. In her late twenties, Linda had given up the meetings, offices, and busy-ness of her business to pursue a new career in therapeutic massage. She wanted more direct contact with people. Linda implemented my program, but she was going through much resistance in getting in touch with what she really wanted.

Some days she felt quite isolated while giving body massages and she yearned for the business world. Other times, she wanted to feel more and

Linda

to discover the treasures of being close and intimate with her clients, as their healing facilitator.

The conflict was enormous. Linda would go into isolation, would not wear her eyeglasses, and would therefore not see for weeks and months on end. Following this isolation, she would wear her weaker therapeutic lens prescription and step out into life once more.

This continued for four years. I remained in partial contact with her and I remember a time in 1985 when she joined one of the weekend seminars I was teaching. A rehabilitative process of the weekend was to explore the fear of blindness. I used music and slides to set the scene and darkened the room. Using blindfolds, I simulated blindness for the participants. The idea was to have them experience what blindness was like, so that when they opened their eyes once again, they could appreciate how much they could really see.

This process touched most of the people in the room, but Linda raised her hand and told us that, six months earlier, her ophthalmologist had diagnosed an incurable disease of her eyes and that she was actually going blind. At first, cloudiness and grayness entered her sight. She could no longer drive but was still facing the future with confidence. Her imminent blindness made Linda experience the "this is it" phenomenon. She couldn't wait for her next vacation, or for next year, to do the things she wanted.

There was no time for her to plan her future vision of seeing. This *was* it! She was preparing to leave for a trip to Europe to visit the museums she had always wanted to see and was planning a trip to California to see the coastline and her relatives. Linda was cramming in as much as she could, providing her eyes and vision with a veritable feast. She was no longer choosing to be a passive victim, saying there was no time or money. This was it. Her life mattered *now*!

Linda's was a rare, progressive eye disease that led to vast amounts of deterioration of the retina. Even though Linda was motivated to help herself, the complementary therapies were started too late and not fully implemented.

A few months later, I visited Linda for a massage. The sensitivity she had developed through her hands performed magic on my chest and around my heart. As a result of her blindness, she had really developed her capacity to feel. Her life continued to be transformed. Linda seized the moment, using her blindness to realize her dream to be closer to people. She chose the oasis. Her daily life became the performance and not just the dress rehearsal.

Facing your resistance can be one of the most frightening steps in discovering the power behind your eyes. Remember the earlier statement about what you want. Now add one that is a little more action-oriented: "With regard to my eyes and vision, what I want is . . . and *to accomplish this my intention is . . ."*

It is the intention that makes a new job, a new relationship, a new home, or giving up contact lenses more of a possibility. What are you really willing to do to make this happen? If you have used your eyes and vision in an unbalanced and nonintegrated way before, begin some Integrated Vision Therapy activities that can shift your old perceptual attitude into a new way of seeing and looking. Here are some steps to follow:

Write down your daily activities and categorize them into whether they involve (1) looking far away (ten feet or beyond) and (2) looking close-up (nine feet to arm's distance).

What is the percentage of time you spend looking in these two ways?

        Far: %   Near: %

If you use contact lenses or eyeglasses, record the number of waking hours you wear them.

Contacts:	hours
Full-strength glasses:	hours
Weaker glasses:	hours
Naked vision:	hours

Note the percentage of time you wear contacts and compare it to the amount of time you wear eyeglasses. What percentage of time do you spend in your naked vision?

If you use contact lenses and you spend more than 50 percent of your time looking at intermediate or close distances, consider wearing eyeglasses designed for 20/40 and wear them for all focused situations. A 20/40 lens prescription gives you about 84 percent clarity and 16 percent blur. Consider a 20/25 pair of eyeglasses or contacts for driving, especially at night or in rainy weather.

If you wear only eyeglasses, follow the same procedures.

If you wear reading glasses, have the prescription cut back so that you have to move objects a little farther away while reading, about four to six inches.

If you don't use eyeglasses or contacts, consider patching one of your eyes. If you experience clarity differences between the eyes, cover the clearer of the two eyes with a patch. If there are no differences in clarity in your naked vision, cover the Harry or Sally eye, depending on which of your perceptions you wish to accentuate.

Some basic guidelines for patching need to be considered: Only wear the patch during non–life-threatening situations. And build up a "wearing time" in fifteen-minute increments, starting with half an hour and not exceeding four consecutive hours. Wearing a patch for longer periods may result in decreased vision fitness of the covered eye. A vision therapist, educator, or behavioral optometrist can suggest additional ways for you to patch. (These professionals can be located through organizations listed in "Resources" at the back of the book.)

I have seen miracles occur from this potent form of Integrated Vision Therapy. Formerly "lazy" eyes begin perceptually to return to life, like a spring flower blossoming in the sun. Your power behind your eyes is turned on, so the sleeping eye, the nerve, and the muscle tissue are restimulated. I have seen people with thick, nearsighted, farsighted, and astigmatic lenses reduce their lens prescriptions by one-third to one-half, and in some cases, set aside their eyeglasses forever.

Susan

Susan, age sixty-nine, had already had one major self-healing experience. She had cured herself of cancer, in spite of a death-sentence from her medical doctor. Only a little farsighted, she became concerned when her ophthalmologist diagnosed a cataract in her left eye. She consulted me in order to begin a home-based Integrated Vision Therapy program to enhance her vision.

At first, Susan covered her right eye with a patch to fully experience her perception through Sally. Many strong feelings emerged. Then, using the Eye-C chart, she began noticing the times when her eyes became immobile and staring. Through breathing and allowing her eyes to move, she accessed her feelings and began seeing more.

Susan increased her vitamin C intake and ate fresh fruit, green leafy vegetables, and sea vegetables such as arame and hijiki (an excellent source of trace minerals). She also visualized the cataract material dissolving. Susan soon discovered more of her own emotional truth and feminine power.

After six months, the fitness of her vision had increased by more than 60 percent (i.e., her perception through the left eye increased). She is now checking with her ophthalmologist to determine if there are also structural changes and improvements in her eye.

When she came to Integrated Vision Therapy, Susan brought strong intention to heal her vision and live a fully productive life. Susan currently works for an agency that helps people deal with their cancer, using her skills and personal experience to empower others with life-threatening diseases. Such empowerment seems to be a key in successfully bringing one's vision into the world.

As explained in chapter 1, a modified lens prescription alters your habitual pattern of *looking* more than *seeing*. Dealing with your intention in life necessitates looking *and* seeing. Creating a little blurring puts you at the edge of your comfort zone. When you slip into moments of visual unconsciousness, the increased blurring will ask you to wake up. Your new state of consciousness requires visual vigilance. A weakened lens prescription allows you to experience the benefits of the blurring/clarity aspects of your naked vision. Strong eyeglasses take away the blur that allows you to see in another dimension.

My blur and double-vision allow me to see energy emanating around my patients' faces. I connect their words with what I see in the measured blur. Spend time in your blur. What do you discover? What can you see differently and create in your home life that will give daily time and space and sharper eyesight? Your reaction to blur is significantly greater than your illusion of how bad your blur is. There are degrees of blur. Learn to not compare the little blur from the weakened lens prescription with the blur customarily experienced without your eyeglasses or contacts. Relax by breathing and blinking.

In my own case, once I began Integrated Vision Therapy I observed the variability of my double vision when some outside influence bothered me, or when I ate inappropriate foods or exercised aerobically. When I became clear and expressed my intention to not live in an unconscious way, the double vision became less frequent. Likewise, if you have blurry vision, you can do this test for yourself using the specially designed Far and Near Eye-C charts. My patients notice their blurry vision varying as their commitment to being clear in their life waxes and wanes.

Sam

Sam expressed his intentions to be more in control of his deteriorating vision, and acquired a 20/40 lens prescription. When I asked him to commit to vision games for fifteen minutes a day, he hesitated. I mentioned that the increased blurring he was experiencing while seeing through his new lenses would bother him more if his intention to bring his clear perceptions to his life was not realized.

Within a couple of months he phoned, complaining the blur was bothering him and that he wanted stronger lenses again.

The blur results from an increased scattering of light over the retina, which calls for more *seeing* of the blind spots in your life. If you are not intent upon dealing with these core issues, the lenses and Integrated Vision Therapy procedures can be bothersome and agitating.

Peter   Peter, an engineer, was in his late forties when he heard about Integrated Vision Therapy. At first he practiced spending time without his thick glasses. He couldn't see the big E on his doctor's eye chart without his glasses. He found a sympathetic vision-therapy optometrist who weakened his glasses. His success was summarized in a letter he wrote to me.

> *I have worn glasses for approximately forty years, and up to about one year ago, I always believed that the only way that I could see properly was through the use of glasses, or to have one of the corneal operations. I have discovered that this is not the case, and that natural procedures exist for improving vision. Furthermore, it can be absolutely exhilarating to experience the process of vision improvement, in particular after being conditioned in the belief that glasses or an operation are the only answer.*
>
> *In my case, my vision one year ago was 20/400, and my glasses had a prescription of –4.50 diopters, complete with bifocals and prisms to compensate for my double vision. I was totally dependent upon my glasses. My current vision is about 20/80 (58.5 percent clearness) to 20/100 (48.9 percent clearness), and the prescription for my glasses is –2.50 diopters, with no prism or bifocals. My eyes are still improving, and I am confident that I will get to a point where I can function almost totally without glasses. I also wish to emphasize that I have not had any operations to my eyes, even though qualified eye doctors have suggested, in the past, that I may need to have an operation to clear up my double vision.*

Peter has since continued making improvements and now there are times during bright sunny periods where he sees well enough to legally drive. This type of improvement in vision is quite common for highly motivated people like Peter. At his last visit, he proudly presented a computerized graph showing the improvement he had achieved.

From a scientific point of view, there are two key variables at play when vision begins to improve. The measurement of the optical variables in the eye, called the refraction, determines the lens prescription to be worn in glasses or contacts. (The refractive power of corrective lenses is measured in diopters, units that increase and decrease in one-quarter steps. The higher the number, the stronger the lens. A plus sign before the number indicates a correction for farsightedness, a minus sign, nearsightedness.) You can think of this as being a measurement of the structure of the eye.

The results of your *looking* at an eye chart like the Eye-C chart indicate your perceptual ability to *see*. This is a functional measurement of your vision and does not necessarily correlate to the structural finding.

In fact, it is normal to see equivalent structural findings between two people, and yet they can have as much as a 60 percent difference in functional eye-chart measurements. This is why you may find your eye doctor invalidating the Eye-C chart improvements in your vision; the eyeball refraction may not have significantly changed. This is very common.

My research findings, now being substantiated in clinical trials by at least thirty other optometrists, indicate the structure of the eye changes much later than chart improvements. Sometimes it takes nine months for the eye measurements to register their first change.

In a double-blind study conducted at Oregon's Pacific University College of Optometry in 1982, an average of 30 percent improvement in eyesight was measured for a group of forty-four people in a three-week Integrated Vision Therapy experimental period. The refractive measurements were recorded and, unlike the perceptual improvements in eyesight, the structural findings were *not* statistically different after three weeks. A control group, whose members underwent the same testing without the treatment, did not show the same statistically significant improvements. Even after they received the identical vision therapy as the experimental group, but without the intensive support, the results remained at a below-significant level. Findings from this study were presented at the 1982 American Academy of Optometry meeting in Chicago, and the study was subsequently published in my book *Seeing Without Glasses*.

Joanne

Joanne's original lens prescription for glasses was –10.50 with –1.25 diopters of astigmatism. She never went without her glasses, since she was unable to wear contacts. She incorporated a home-based Integrated Vision Therapy, and after four years, the astigmatism was gone and the measured nearsightedness was down to –5.00. These were actual structural changes, verified by an optometrist who was not administering the vision therapy program. Joanne had also reduced her wearing of glasses by 85 percent.

It is usual for individuals with degrees of nearsightedness and astigmatism less than Joanne's to be totally out of glasses once the vision therapy has been integrated into their life, as they have fewer dioptric filters—lenses that hide the perceptual truth of the past—to remove from the front of their eyes. In cases of farsightedness, the dioptric measurements can be reduced faster, depending on the person's age. Beyond age forty, the process is a little more complicated because of the changes in near vision. Clinical evidence suggests that vision therapy can improve visual function. The accrued benefits prevent future structural distortions and disease, when the practices are continued on a daily basis.

It is easy to get caught up in just trying to understand the numerical changes of the optic variables while practicing Integrated Vision Therapy. But remember, your true purpose is to integrate new ways of *seeing* into your life. Understand what your eyes are attempting to tell you. Rest your eyes, breathe, and stay present. Work on *seeing* through your heart. Practice *looking* at everything in your life with kindness. This is the most profound way to create the best results.

Surrendering to Fear

One of my greatest fears in life was opening myself to being vulnerable. My professional training had schooled me to be the invincible healer. I was not to expose my humanness or my emotional fragility.

By my mid-thirties I had, in a sense, reached the pinnacle of my career in clinical optometry and academics. Yet I felt empty, my heart was shut off, and I yearned for a different way of relating to people and to life.

I began surrounding myself with acquaintances and friends who were willing to honestly share their perceptions of me. My double vision was lessening, but I still needed to free the power of my intuition, creativity, and heart connection.

I further modified my eating and enjoyed the ritual of preparing food. Believing that red meat is not a healthy food, I had been following a vegetarian diet, but as I listened and felt what my body needed, I utilized my knowledge of healthy eating in a less restricted way and included organic meat and wild game in my diet. Consuming food became a ceremony of celebration and nurturing. I sought out bodyworkers who, through massage, structural manipulation, and acupressure, allowed me to unlock the physical gates of my muscles.

I deepened my understanding of the relationship between my emotional states, my perception, and my scoliosis (curvature of the spine). I had vision therapists direct me through experiential processes where I could no longer deny my distorted perceptions. One of the most powerful experiences occurred in the office of retired optometrist Robert Pepper.

Dr. Pepper had an Olympic-size trampoline in his office. During the sixth session of a twelve-session program, I was jumping on the trampoline while he flashed five-number sequences on a screen at speeds varying from 1/10 of a second to 1/250 of a second. I called out the sequence of numbers that I saw as I bounced. I was obtaining an 80 percent correct response until Dr. Pepper flashed a sequence while my feet were still on the trampoline, as opposed to being in the air. This variation from the routine upset my perceptions in such a way that I saw the numbers slanted at an oblique angle. My personality took control, and I asked Dr. Pepper to focus the projector. He said he hadn't changed the focus.

The experience was very humbling, and I realized that, in a moment of distress and feeling out of control, I had distorted my perception along the same oblique direction of my astigmatism. This feedback was worth the whole program. I collapsed onto the mat, and after feeling intently for a while, I made a commitment to seeing the truth. I reclaimed my power and vowed to observe the future distortions in my vision, or the way I *see* life.

Fear freezes us in our tracks. We see the flashing red and blue lights, the perspiration starts, and we become like children who have to face the principal. Instead of being accountable and taking responsibility for our actions, we may deny our actions and try to talk our way out of the situation. If we are successful, we pat our personality on the back and speed off again into life.

Looking at specific markings in a patient's iris one day, I began to count all the possible variations of fear: abandonment, separation, rejection, loss of love, poverty, punishment, assault, change, abuse, darkness, blindness, demons, falling, insanity, humiliation, mistakes, failure, and death. It is amazing how fear can dominate our perceptions and affect our lives. Susan Jeffer's book *Feel the Fear and Do It Anyway* has helped many of us to consider fear in a new light. I teach my patients a process that deepens this idea.

Place your index and middle fingers under your wrist to find your pulse. Now, consider the list of fears above and choose the one thing you fear the most. A common fear my patients share is fear of separation or loss of love. As you feel the fear, does your pulse vary? Note the change and then consider something exciting in your life; feel again for changes. Usually there is no significant change between the pulse levels of fear and excitement, which suggests that our bodies don't know the difference. Only our personality, or survival state, knows the difference.

The healing power is the switch in our mind that makes us able to generate a feeling of excitement instead of fear. Seize a negative event as an opportunity rather than a crisis. The shift in our perceptions stimulates this inner transformation.

Carol   Carol saw her life in two distinct parts: her desire to pursue her career as a teacher of drama and theater at the university, and her desire to maintain her primary relationship with her live-in lover of ten years. The intensity of focus needed for her career stretched the balance between these two desires. The first hint of breakdown for Carol had occurred ten years previously, when one day her body sent a warning signal called Bell's palsy. A major nerve from the brain was paralyzed, and the whole left side of Carol's face froze. Carol, aged thirty-five, performed the necessary first-aid steps to handle the crisis—she sought out medical diagnoses and got more rest. But her recent move across the country and the excitement of her then-new relationship precluded her from making any "life-changing" decisions. Her crisis would need to return in the form of another emergency situation before Carol would understand the significance of her body's message. She herself acknowledged her incredible *need* to act and teach. The idea of slowing down or stopping terrified her.

Carol's farsightedness and astigmatism manifested as blurring along the perceptual meridian of spiritual communication. She had subconsciously made a choice to block the spiritual part of her existence, substituting work, work, and more work to fulfill her inner longings. But why? What was she avoiding? This would only be revealed ten years later when the "rubber hit the road." Her physical brakes were applied when she experienced double vision, mostly at distances of eight feet or beyond. Her dependency upon eyeglasses began to increase. Her "gift" of an illness was a diagnosis of myasthenia gravis, an eye disease with little or no available treatment at the time. Her double vision was most disturbing and inconvenient. Her partner had to drive her fifteen miles to and from work. The message her body was giving her finally became clear to Carol. She had to stop and reevaluate her life.

Through my interaction with Carol, she began to see how her astigmatism was screaming for her to pay more attention to her physical and spiritual well-being. Her farsightedness was a rebellious pushing outward of her personality that focused beyond her internal self to her career and achievement. Soon after we began Integrated Vision Therapy, Carol chose to take a nine-month sabbatical in order to initiate a deep healing transformation within herself. At last, she paid attention to her body and its deep inner messages. For the first time ever, she allowed others to assist her. She activated her own power behind her eyes by allowing herself to receive love and support from five significant people in her life. Carol surrendered to the fear of going blind and being incapacitated. From this place of understanding, a new and balanced lifestyle evolved. Miraculously, her double vision began fusing into healthier single vision as she integrated a unified perception of her work and personal life into her daily existence.

My first experience in converting fear to excitement occurred when my daughter was five years old. One day we visited a fairground together. As we walked around looking at the different rides and amusements, Julia pointed to a slide, saying she wanted to go on it. It seemed a relatively tame activity, so I held her tightly and down we went. Repeating the slide run a few times whet her appetite for more adventurous play. She pointed to a faster, and, as I perceived it, more dangerous ride for a five-year-old, and one she would have to go on by herself. I caught myself saying no, realizing that Julia was experiencing excitement and that I was fearing her falling out and being hurt.

I was focused on the half-empty glass! I switched my perceptual process and said okay. She hung on for dear life, screaming and having a terrific time. I remembered a time when I was eight years old, when my mother needed to get me off a ride just like this one because I was vomiting. As I opened to this connection, I felt my fear subsiding and I became captivated by Julia's excitement. A year later, Julia and I visited Disneyland and I promised myself we would exclude no rides. I wanted to dive into my fears and transform them into excitement, and we did!

Chapter 5

The Challenge
To Be Clear

Seeing within changes one's outer vision.

—Joseph Chilton Pearce

People need a sense of safety, a place where they can let down their walls and defenses and talk about what's really going on in their lives without fear that anyone is going to judge or reject them.

—Dr. Dean Ornish

Visual Noise

We as human beings pay a price for the astounding technology we have created. Via television networks like CNN, we are able to watch firsthand accounts of world strife right in our living rooms. Computers allow us to travel, via electronic bulletin boards, all over the world and talk to our fellow world citizens. Video games give children a way to develop their hand-eye coordination. The bad news is that our eyes are not biologically designed for long periods of any of these activities. We can develop eyestrain, and if this persists, any predisposition for nearsightedness, farsightedness, or astigmatism is accelerated. The number of people seeking help for their eyes and vision has grown significantly over the last ten years.

It is easy to slip into a sort of "unconsciousness" when watching television or working at a computer. Children playing video games or watching movies seem to be in a hypnotic trance. The eye muscles can become locked in their focus, resulting in symptoms of blurry vision and tired, burning, and watering eyes. The repetitive nature of most electronic devices creates a one-focus mind-set. Over time, this produces a form of mind habituation, and our vision sense becomes dull.

The eyes must move in order for vision to be stimulated, but for most of us our modern world is full of too much visual stimulation. Have you noticed how tired you feel after visiting a busy supermarket or shopping mall? The typical shopping-related visual environment is designed to catch your attention. Your conscious vision is unable to cope with so much visual stimulation, or "visual noise."

The same visual assault occurs in large cities, in work environments, and sadly, in schools. In most cases, a schoolchild's eyes are overloaded with visual stimulation from books, blackboards, video monitors, and microfiche. The natural reaction is to shut down the foveal vision and stop looking, but the challenge is that the seeing retina is still being bombarded with much of that visual noise, so we may still feel exhausted. Contrast this type of stimulation with that in nature, where the eyes can gently wander over green vegetation, running water, and sandy or rugged or rolling terrain stopping to focus on whatever peaks our interest at the moment. This natural way of using our eyes supports the integrity of visual function.

The same visual noise that promotes the shutting down of foveal vision can be used constructively. If we are willing to take some responsibility, we can protect our eyes and vision and not have to give up our computers, television, and video games. Taking frequent breaks and practicing vision games can stimulate relaxation and encourage high-level vision fitness.

When you feel your mind wandering and your eyes becoming tired, sleepy, or burning, take a break. When using your eyes in high-tech visual environments, you might even set a timer for thirty and sixty minutes. This alarm system will be a reminder to take that break. Your eyes will love the rest. When the alarm signals, cover your eyes and palm them for at least five full and connected breaths.

I am personally thankful for this visual noise now that I am more conscious of the sensitivity of my eyes and vision. Prior to working on a computer, I hardly ever stopped during the day to breathe or cover my eyes with my hands. I now frequently leave my desk to stretch my body, and look out a window. Try this yourself: Let your mind leave the job at hand and take an imaginary holiday to Greece: warm sand, hot sun, and relaxation for your face and eyes. After palming, spend a moment looking into the distance, preferably out a window. Let your attention and focus go far off into the distance and contemplate summertime, vacation, swimming, and fun.

Back at the computer screen, let your eyes play a shifting game every thirty minutes: Place brightly colored stickers on the four corners of the monitor or screen. Imagine your eyes are like a bug that can hop from one corner to the other. As you shift, breathe and enjoy the motion. As long as your eyes are moving, they are under less strain and you will not be tempted to try to see anything. Again, look out and beyond the immediate area of near-space into the distance.

Your eyes and the conditions of disease or wellness present opportunities to grow as a person. Treat the Integrated Vision Therapy as a rite of passage to a higher level of consciousness. Problems are transformed into challenges, and the element of excitement is added to your daily life journey. The result is more power and illumination from within.

Observe your daily life for automatic behavior. Do you follow the same routine? If so, your vision needs stimulation, a change of pace. The creative part of your mind can generate solutions to end any habitual patterning. The vision games you are learning are a creative way for you to restore balanced ways of looking (doing) and seeing (being) in your life.

Why have we, as a culture, created a world of visual noise? How do these outside distractions contribute and take away from our essence? Consider how visual noise has disrupted the traditional family. It is not uncommon for children to have their own televisions in their bedrooms. Their visual sensing is smothered with information about unnecessary things to buy. Family members used to spend hours sharing clan tales. Skills were passed down through stories, families participated in activities around the home and together they cultivated the land and grew crops. Hunting, building homes, and spending time outdoors stimulated the eyes and vision.

Now we feel we have good reason to be wary of spending too much time outdoors: the sun could damage our skin, our children may be kidnapped, or we could be mugged by a stranger. Our perceptions have taken on a defensive posture. We feel a need to protect ourselves from the salesperson, the canvasser at the front door, or the beggar on the street. This way of being sets up the autonomic nervous system to act in a defensive way. The fight-or-flight response sets in, and the function of our eyes is controlled by a nervous system that is working in response to fear. This pulls the balance toward the personality part of your mind.

When people perceive the world to be unfriendly, they imagine outside forces attacking them. The former enemy was the wild animal. Today it is rush-hour traffic, the neighbor's barking dog, a blaring stereo. These perceptions exacerbate the feeling of being alone and battling a world of enemies. Your perceptions are numbed by the visual noise, and your eyes begin to see from a fearful "victim" position.

Reclaim your power as a human being by using integrated breathing.

Acknowledge how your life is aided by the modern-day conveniences, but spend some time *not* watching television, reading, or working on a computer. Walk in nature, look at a river, lake, or ocean, or hike a mountain. Bring varied experiences to your eyes. Feel the power of nature charging your "vision batteries." Give your soul a chance to peer out when next confronted by the noise of your visual world. Every moment is an opportunity to stimulate and relax your vision.

Dolly came to me seeking help for her nearsightedness. From an extensive intake interview and examination we found that the onset of Dolly's nearsightedness concurred with her parents' divorce more than twenty years previously. The divorce had left Dolly feeling torn between her two parents. Following the divorce Dolly became overly focused on independence. She also vowed to one day have a wonderful husband and family.

Dolly

A therapist, Dolly was now at an age where she felt culturally pressured to be married and have children. Seeing her friends with their families made her feel uneasy about her own future. Dolly had secured an education and purchased her own home. Now she had visions of starting on a new path by opening a private practice and working from her home.

Dolly had been in and out of relationships, but when she met Gary she felt she had found a man who could share her soul in marriage. There were complications, however. Gary was married with two small children. As is usual in the early stages of a new relationship, the fire of the courtship blinded Dolly to the difficulty of the situation. Gary promised to divorce his wife and marry Dolly, but he had to support his two daughters and was on a limited income. Dolly desperately wanted to have a man she could love and take care of, and she feared she might not find the man of her life in time to bear children. She invited Gary to move in with her (although he and his wife were still not divorced), because he didn't have enough money for his own place. Now the space in Dolly's house that was to be her new office was occupied with Gary's possessions, including a queen-size waterbed. All her dreams of self-employment came second to the relationship.

Gary was now quite comfortable in his new home. Dolly's vision progress stalled. Gary proposed marriage and presented Dolly with a diamond ring. Dolly loved Gary and felt she had found her soulmate, yet during the next six months she grew more and more frustrated.

The fitness of Dolly's vision remained the same through her weaker 20/40 lens prescription, and she had not made any headway with her new career. The lack of increased vision clarity despite the vision-therapy lens prescription was the indicator she needed. Dolly realized that her soul was asking her for a change. She needed to step into her power and *see* the reality of what she had created. Once Dolly reclaimed her vision clarity, she moved very fast. She asked Gary to move out, waterbed and all!

Dolly's visual progress sped up and she has truly taken control of her life—which still includes Gary, but in a partnership where they are both independently strong.

Dolly's story illustrates the benefit of seeking balance between our personal desires for relationships and careers. The visual noise we create in our lives, and the addictions we begin to see, can serve as a red light warning us to recover balance between the doing and being parts of our lives.

Seeing Your Addictions

Our visual world has become saturated with things. We produce tons of items that crowd our homes, offices, and cities. The materialistic world cries out: Look at me! We focus outside of ourselves, fixating on our careers, relationships, and the things we can buy to satisfy our fearful personalities. The modern prescription for health and happiness is to stuff ourselves full of processed food, cover our bodies with synthetic garments, and surround ourselves with junk. How we look has become more important than how we feel. Designer clothes, cosmetics, imported luxury cars, and large homes are the illusions of success. If the pressure to have all of this is an illusion, what is reality? In a true Zen fashion, a teacher once said to me, "Spend a few years contemplating these questions":

- At the end of the day, what brings you peace of mind?
- What aspects of your life connect you to your soul?
- Where in your daily living do you put pressure on yourself to have certain material things?
- In a typical day and week of your life, where do you experience being joyous and full of light?
- What in the outside world do you need to possess in order to feel empowered?
- Where do you give your power away?

Anne Wilson Schaef, in her landmark book *When Society Becomes an Addict,* questions whether our lifestyles and unresolved issues lead to addictive patterns of behavior. Perhaps looking outside ourselves for the solutions to our life problems is a form of visual addiction. Prolonged external foveal fixation ("looking for the answer") leads to eye and mind fatigue. It is hard work to focus outward. As you master integrated breathing and watching a candle flame, you will notice how much more relaxing it is to look inward. Soul-seeing is less fatiguing than searching for answers through your survival-based personality. The intention of Integrated Vision Therapy is to allow you to *see* more often through filters of your soul and less often through your personality.

Your eyes are designed to focus on life in an effortless way, which requires moving them. One of my favorite vision games is "Becoming Shifty-Eyed." While looking at the Far or Near Eye-C chart, begin moving your eyes from letter to letter, like stepping from one stone to the next while crossing a stream.

Practice this exercise now. Let your eyes dance around, stopping at different points on the Eye-C chart as you become proficient at shifting. Practice using the chart this way while you talk on the telephone.

While engaged in conversation with a friend, let your eyes dance from their eyes to their nose, ears, eyebrows, mouth, and cheeks. Notice if your ability to do this changes your focus. Breathe and blink. Begin to feel relaxed while you negotiate your world. It is not necessary for you to live in a cave in order to free yourself from the pressure to see! Bring these Integrated Vision Therapy principles into your awareness. Each time you break your habitual way of *looking*, you are firing up your power. Enjoy the benefits of balanced vision as you peel away your strong lenses and your eyes, brain, and mind relax during the day. As you become relaxed and clear in your mind, celebrate your new perceptions of the challenges you face in your life.

Using the following list as a guide, observe how you use your eyes during the day in these situations:

- Traveling to work
- Driving a car
- Sitting at a desk
- Conversing with people
- Being with your children
- Reading
- Watching television
- Using a computer
- Talking on the telephone

What are your eyes revealing to you? What addictive patterns keep you speeding down the road, busy with your *doing* life and missing the beauty around you? An addiction is a pattern of behavior that is played out in your life in order to protect your feelings. Selling out your soul is another form of addiction. Identify and write down your addictive patterns and then ask the question again: "What do I want?" Honor your truth for your life.

In vision care, the greatest addiction is the indiscriminate prescribing of strong eyeglasses. It is unfortunate that most optometrists and ophthalmologists have not been sensitized to the idea that eyeglasses are an addictive device. Most people for whom eyeglasses are prescribed end up needing stronger lens prescriptions the second time their eyes are examined. They are then in the grip of the next greatest addiction: blind acceptance of a prescription lens as the only solution to a vision problem. You have probably been told to wear your glasses because they will "correct your vision." What the doctor is really saying is that the lenses will *compensate* for your blurry vision.

An artificial lens is a prescription from an optometrist or optician. The potency of a prescribed drug is carefully regulated to keep you from becoming addicted to the substance. Isn't it time for you to question the potency of the lens prescriptions that sit in front of your eyes? Prescription glasses that are too strong create an addictive illusion of the world as being perfectly clear.

I believe that for most people, strong eyeglasses enforce a limited, nonmultidimensional state of vision. Your strong lens prescriptions keep your soul suppressed. Your focus on the material, foveal, logical plane dominates your vision. Your emotional, feeling, heart-connected perceptions begin to suffer. Your two-eyed vision disintegrates, and the separation between your soul- and personality-related perceptions is deepened. This happens to wake you up to the need to see beyond the physical parameters that you think are possible. Two-eyed vision is a stepping stone to higher levels of seeing where the soul and personality become further integrated.

The originating force behind the development of Integrated Vision Therapy was the lens prescription. After ten years of observing the need to increase lens prescriptions for patients, I decided to introduce a well-established two-eyed testing method. Even though the two-eyed system of examining is taught in most doctoral programs in vision therapy, few optometrists actually test with both eyes open at the same time. They usually cover one eye and test the open one. In my experience, this form of testing is unnatural and leads to unnecessarily strong prescriptions. I found this out during my first years in practice when I recognized that in a significant number of cases the strong compensating lens prescription that I routinely prescribed for full-time wear induced a disruption in two-eyed vision. I realized that *my* addiction to having my patients see perfectly clearly would, in the long-term, result in *their* addiction to wearing continually stronger glasses.

Then serendipity knocked on my door. A patient named Saul asked me one day if I knew anything about eye exercises for improving vision. He was committed to helping his eyes, because each year the doctor gave him a new, stronger prescription for nearsightedness. I mentioned my research findings on the disruption of two-eyed vision, and we agreed to investigate whether a weaker lens prescription might help Saul's eyes get stronger. We reduced his lens prescription from –8.00 to –6.00. The first amazing result was that the weaker lens prescription allowed Saul's eyes to integrate. Again using the two-eye testing method, I was able to examine the right eye while the left eye participated only slightly. The reduced lens prescription decreased the stress upon the two eyes so that the brain and mind could more efficiently unite the vision from both eyes. Anatomically, the Harry and Sally foveas were in a more harmonious relationship.

The incoming light became more evenly distributed over Saul's entire retina, enabling him to focus his mind more accurately and to integrate his perceptions. Saul commented on how comfortable the weaker eyeglasses felt, even though his distance vision was a little blurry. He felt like an addict who had been weaned from his substance. The weaker lens prescription gave him enough vision to legally drive, and he felt empowered. He was breaking his habit of wearing stronger eyeglasses.

I received a phone call from Saul ten days later. He said his vision seemed very clear through the new eyeglasses. I tested his eyes and found that he could use a new weaker lens prescription of –5.00. Saul had, in a short time, accessed his own internal power of 1.00 diopter. Visually he could now reach three feet farther into life; that is, he could see three feet farther away. I asked him if he felt different. Saul said his career had taken a twist; he had accepted a challenging new assignment and felt very self-assured about this decision.

This clinical success was the beginning of my fifteen-year research journey. Clinical trials involving tens of thousands of people have convinced me and other optometrists of the addictive nature of most compensating lenses. If you are open-minded and committed to strengthening and integrating your vision, a weaker lens prescription is a viable and practical way for you to wean yourself from your addictive past. The weaker lens prescription is a natural biofeedback device that helps you monitor your perceptions. When you *see* through the filters of the addictive personality, your vision will be more blurry. If you use integrated breathing, allowing you to relax and enter your heart, your soul-vision will be clearer.

Dis-ease Leads to Disease

Allopathic medicine focuses on the presence of disease. Some bug, virus, or bacteria has invaded your body and that is why you are sick. There is an equivalent form of allopathic vision care: "Your eyeball is long, short, or warped, and this is why you need glasses. You are getting old, and this is why you must wear reading glasses. For your age, it is normal to have floaters. For your degree of nearsightedness, it is common to have retinal detachments. The depleted ozone layer is why you have cataracts at age thirty-five. Your eye turns in because the muscle is weak." Very seldom does an optometrist or ophthalmologist consider that the person may have been involved in the genesis of their disease.

Studies have shown that if you imagine terrible things happening in your life, the flow of blood to the heart decreases. In a landmark study on heart disease, physician Dean Ornish has demonstrated that the buildup of fatty plaque in heart patients' arteries can be reversed when they make a complete and challenging lifestyle change. In *Dr. Ornish's Program for Reversing Heart Disease*, he notes that although the heart is universally recognized as the seat of human compassion, spirit, and love, cardiologists never discuss the heart in these terms. Ornish, however, encourages patients to imagine the wellness of their hearts. He maintains that many people are in pain, spiritually and emotionally, and that illnesses of the heart stem from being withdrawn. He feels that perceptions of competition, or emotions such as excessive self-involvement, hostility, and cynicism, can unleash hormones that lead to a constriction of the arteries.

Is it possible that, in the same way, your eye condition is a manifestation of unskillful perceptions? By unskillful, I mean that you do not know how to integrate your perceptions of soul and personality. Perhaps long before your condition was diagnosed there were subtle signs of dis-ease. Twitches, frowning, periods of blurry vision, momentary pains, and loss of peripheral side vision may have been precursors to your eye problem. I am suggesting that the onset of disease or eye problems follows a developmental continuum over time. Dis-ease precedes disease. You don't suddenly wake up one day with a disease of the eyes. We expose ourselves to disease by our ill-adapted lifestyles.

The most poignant example is the case of glaucoma. By definition, this condition is associated with a buildup of pressure in the eye, and it is often associated with high blood pressure. But ophthalmologists seldom connect the presence of glaucoma with pressure in the patient's *life*. If they do, they may simply suggest that the patient needs to lead a more sedentary lifestyle.

The way you set up your daily living, whether it be a fast-paced doing, or a more even-keeled being, will modify the state of your nervous system. Your autonomic nervous system is attempting to seek balance. Its primary aim is to preserve the integrity of your endocrine system, as well as to ensure that your heart and breathing patterns are able to conserve energy. Aches, pains, burning, fatigue, and sleepiness of the eyes are subtle communication signals of dis-ease and beginning signs of imbalance. The prudent approach is to learn to read these signals and thus avoid the next step of disease. Why wait until the disease shows up on your doorstep? Practice looking deeply at your eye symptoms, *seeing* when they appear, and noticing any emotional and/or physical reasons for their appearance. This exercise necessitates being clear and truthful with yourself. You will find that integrated breathing, candle-watching, and nose- and eye crossing and uncrossing are good vision games to play prior to introspective self-exploration. Are you willing to be fully accountable for your unskillful *looking* and *seeing* of the events in your life? If you are, then Integrated Vision Therapy will make a difference in your life.

Dr. Smith

A recent consultation with Dr. Smith, a podiatrist, reminded me of what happens when we ignore the significance of dis-ease, and how important it is to be clear when checking out different treatment options. Dr. Smith had a long history of nearsightedness, for which he compensated for many years with eyeglasses. Like Stephen, whom I mentioned earlier, Dr. Smith was lured by the quick and easy approach offered by laser surgery to eliminate his nearsightedness. He didn't consider that his eye condition was a form of dis-ease. If he better understood why the condition was present, he might have seized the opportunity to grow personally instead. As it turned out, he needed a bigger and later wake-up call to capture his attention.

Dr. Smith's nearsightedness and astigmatism, measuring –6.00, was mainly in his left eye. The situation began when he was a young boy; and represented the distorted way his eyes recorded what was happening in his life. Although I cannot disclose details of the events that were taking place at that time, it would appear that Dr. Smith reacted incongruently through his right and left eyes. While he preserved his ability to see far through the logical, right-eye side of his being, he shrank in his left-eye side associated with feelings, creativity, and intuition. Had someone been able to help him understand the meaning of the incident from the perspective of soul essence, his perceptual response would have been less visually reactive, i.e., more skillful and integrated, with less likelihood of his eyeball warping. Instead, the young boy was encouraged to wear eyeglasses, which hid the vital message that his intellect needed to fully merge with his intuition to lead to integrated vision and a harmonizing of soul and personality.

Unless there is an integration of the two perceptual channels of the eyes, an imbalance exists between the intellectual and intuitive parts of our being. This can lead to the personality having to dominate and protect us. The name of the game is then survival. If ever-stronger lenses continue to mask the blurring of our past, we cannot fully reach higher levels of integration. Because Dr. Smith's vision was naturally clearer through his right eye, his logical and rational side dominated his view of life. From a family-tree perspective, had his mother provided dominant influences and executed this power in his early life, he might have made perceptual, and ultimately visual, choices to further develop this rational "male" side of his being.

The lower vision fitness in Dr. Smith's left eye remained for forty years, at which time he underwent the laser surgery, first on the left and then on the right eye. Shortly after the right-eye procedure, Dr. Smith's left eye developed a retinal tear, which resulted in significant floaters. Finally he got the message that he needed to pay attention to what his eyes were revealing to him. Although the surgery offered great hope of correcting his vision imbalances, the bigger and more life-threatening problem of floaters surfaced. Dr. Smith made a number of positive lifestyle changes; however, the resulting distorted vision was so intense that he had to cease practicing podiatry.

Dr. Smith chose not to pursue Integrated Vision Therapy. His situation humbly reminds me to pay attention to all the dis-eases in my life. When I acknowledge my difficulties, I feel clearer. Can you look at your dis-ease and continue challenging yourself to be clear?

Chapter 6

What You Say Is
What You See!

*Look into all things without prejudice and you will see into
the very nature of what you are looking at.*

—from the Flowering Light Tantra,
an ancient story from
the Tibetan Dür Bön tradition

To Listen Is to Be Liberated

The way you speak about yourself is the way you *see* your life in
your mind. Interference in eyesight, whether it be a refractive situation or a disease of the eye, can often be traced to self-defeating
language, both internalized and spoken aloud. Vision disturbances are your
eyes expressing your doubts and fears. In this chapter, we will probe how
what you say becomes what you see! If you discover that what you say is
not what you wish to see, you can restructure your mental vision. As you
become clear, your eyesight will display the compelling clarity of your
language.

The way we verbalize our thoughts is an area of great fascination for
me. As I developed my own vision I began listening to myself speak. Much
of my communication was laced with negative impressions. I was shocked
to discover that my mind was so filled with cynical thoughts. No wonder I
was so judgmental of what I saw in my life. One of my father's favorite
sayings was: "Why don't you see the bright side of things?" How can we
see clearly when our thoughts are jaded with distorted perceptions? The
first step is to listen to ourselves talk.

I found this difficult. Since I was already a public speaker, I began tape
recording my lectures. When video technology became available, I began
video recording my presentations and would intently listen to how I phrased
my thoughts. I realized that, as with training my vision, I needed to employ mental discipline in order to speak with clarity. I listened to my telephone conversations more closely. I heard myself saying: "I don't know, I

can't, I hope, I'll try, maybe sometime, later." I was also projecting lots of blame, insinuating that the world "out there" was responsible for my misfortunes.

My greatest challenge was in casual conversation. This is where I heard myself lapse into "negative self-talk." When I relaxed with friends, I reverted to an undisciplined way of speaking. I recognized that my speech lacked focus and intention. This imaged my uncentered way of *looking* at life. (Recall that I had double vision, and my challenge was to learn to cross my eyes.) I would start a project, such as reading a book, and invariably would get only three-quarters of the way through before quitting. Making the connection between my mind, the way I saw things, and what was happening in my life was a revelation.

The French clinician Dr. Alfred Tomatis, a pioneer in auditory perception, has documented that our listening can be affected by emotional events in our lives. Dr. Tomatis analyzes the audiogram, the record of a patient's hearing capabilities, in such a way that he can pinpoint the period in which trauma may have occurred. As in vision therapy, where a distinction is made between sight and vision, Dr. Tomatis points out that our ability to hear something doesn't necessarily mean we have the full capacity to listen. The dips in the audiogram reflect an emotional reason for not listening. Dr. Tomatis superimposes sophisticated therapeutic sounds over classical music, to which his patients listen. With time, the patients are able to learn more effectively, read faster, learn second and third languages, and sing.

Reconsider the principle of holism: every part of your being is a microcosm of the whole. A thought, a casual statement, or an inconsequential glance probably affects many parts of your brain. Your goal is to integrate these elements of your total being into new perceptions and alertness. In this way, you can access your power and bring this clarity directly to your eyes.

I recall listening to songs as a youngster. I would hear the words but couldn't remember them. While practicing eye crossing, I trained myself to listen and hear, an exercise demanding concentration similar to the concentration I needed to implement vision therapy. I soon began remembering words to the songs. As my vision became integrated, my ability to recall deepened. Listening to vocals became a pleasurable activity; I kept visualizing the magnificence of the many networks of nerve pathways between the hearing parts of my brain and my vision.

This whole-person training will impact your life in numerous ways.

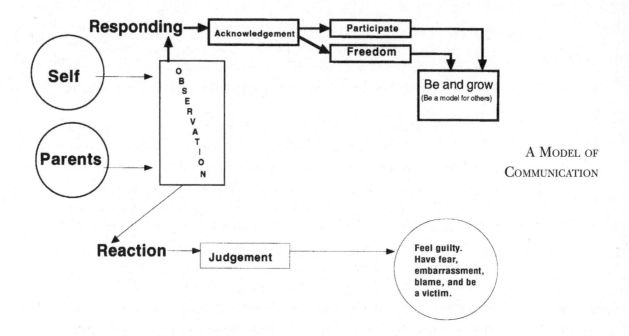

Your reading and language will become more fluid. What you hear, think, say, and see will become congruent. Listening to yourself teaches you to pay attention to what you see. This process deepens your intuition and the way you relate through your senses.

When you don't see clearly, you don't hear as well. But clear vision coupled with a discerning ear enables you to be compassionate through your senses. This integration is the highest form of being. Practice listening while holding a loving feeling and focused vision. The next time someone is talking, look at him or her with the warmhearted feeling you generated through the candle-watching and integrated breathing. Then add the next dimension of listening: Attempt to see past all judgments and your analysis of what the person is saying. Listen for the way, within every communication, that the person is asking to be loved. Notice whether you have an urge to let words slip out of your mouth while you are listening to the person speak.

If you catch yourself thinking while listening, stop, take an integrated breath, and connect with the person's eyes. Feel yourself returning to your heart. Integrated breathing encourages you to feel calmness. This process produces stillness. As you relax, listen and let go of mental and physical tension.

Through stillness, you can also simply learn to be with yourself. Hear the wind, the water, and other movements of nature. Learn to listen without prejudice, then you can *see* with discernment. To see with discernment means to let go of judgments and prejudice, and to lessen the effects of your core beliefs. To have vision this clear, you must have an open heart. Feel and see what is. Here is an exercise you can use to encourage this experience.

Choose either the Far or the Near Eye-C chart and position yourself at a distance where you can see half the letters without your glasses or contacts. Take a few integrated breaths and blink every three seconds. Relax your shoulders and do a few head rotations, first clockwise, then counterclockwise. Feel your shoulders and neck muscles relaxing as you move your head. Then record your baseline level of vision—the smallest letters you can read without straining.

Next, think of a situation in your life in which you feel challenged. This could be your health, a relationship, your eyes, money, family, or career. Once you have a clear picture in your mind and/or a feeling in your body, create a statement that describes your situation. Here are a few examples of situations and descriptions that my patients have shared with me.

> *Career:* I hate my job. My boss gets on my nerves. My supervisor is a pain.
>
> *Primary relationship:* I hold myself back. I am afraid my wife is going to walk out. I feel stuck. I am unhappy in my marriage. I want out of my relationship.
>
> *Money:* I never seem to have enough money. Money is tight. My paycheck doesn't last.
>
> *Health:* I don't digest food very well. My body is full of aches and pains. I am weak.
>
> *Eyes:* My eyes are not working well. I need to fix them. I am getting old.
>
> *Family:* I never see my mother. My father is a tyrant. I am not very close to my parents.

Keep searching your soul until you have two or three sentences that describe your situation. While looking at the Eye-C chart, say each sentence aloud. Pause for a moment and observe whether your perception of the letters changes with each statement.

There are three possible responses. The clarity or darkness of the letters may stay the same, they may get clearer or darker, or you may find the chart becoming more blurry. Note your perceptual response with each sentence. Changes in clarity demonstrate the power of language in molding your perceptions. This exercise can be repeated whenever you wish to explore your feelings about a given situation. Each time you repeat the exercise, the new level of *seeing* the situation becomes the next baseline.

I find that many of my patients have difficulty in what I call "seeing below the throat." For many, *seeing* is a mental activity rather than a whole-body experience. That mental activity is actually *looking*. Seeing demands feeling. You will probably find that certain statements cause a marked, blurry change in your perceptions. These are the ones to focus on. Your goal is to create a sentence that has the opposite meaning—a positive expression of feeling—that can help you determine what is true and what may be required to deal with the situation. For example, if you say you love your job and that simply does not feel right, then you may need to reevaluate your work choices. The therapeutic value of continually repeating the positive state-ment is the deeper feeling that emerges. For example, saying "I have all the money I need," may at first feel patently untrue. The next time you prac-tice the exercises, anger or frustration may surface. A while later, the same anxiety may move you into action to bring more money to you. Soon a new career opportunity becomes apparent.

Here are some examples of positive statements applied to our previous example.

Career: I enjoy my job. My boss is stimulating. I feel compassion toward my supervisor.

Primary relationship: I am reaching out. I am communicating my fears about my wife leaving the marriage. I am becoming clear. My marriage is allowing me to grow. I am choosing to stay in this relationship.

Money: I have all the money I need. When I am creative, I have money. My paycheck provides enough money for my needs.

Health: My digestion is improving. My body tells me what it needs, and I listen. I am strong.

Eyes: My eyes are learning to see. I am nurturing them. I am gaining wis-dom.

Family: I am reaching out to my mother. Father is a challenge. I am open to reaching out to my family.

The more you talk positively about yourself, your life, and your per-sonal vision, the better are your chances for improving your visual func-tion. Merely being able to hear something does not mean you understand it. Likewise, just because you see something, such as the words on this page, does not guarantee that you have internalized the full intent of the idea. Understanding full intent requires full vision. Only when you are fully present and mindful of every action are you reaching for the power behind your eyes. If you allow your personality to sneak in for one moment, or if you slip into thinking, you may lose the intuitive experience of *knowing*. Language affects your perceptions in the same way. If you think and speak in a pessimistic way, you are programming your vision and eyes to see in the same manner.

Giving my patients feedback about their spoken words has proved to be a most effective aspect of Integrated Vision Therapy. Most people are amazed at their sloppy language. At first I audiotaped our sessions so that they could review the way they spoke during our time together. I deepened this process by eventually videotaping our consultations. I would ask my patients specific questions and later review the video segments with them. We listened to their language and also watched their facial and eye gestures during various responses.

The video picture provided me with superb feedback about the differences between their Harry and Sally perceptions. Sometimes I would turn off the sound and simply watch the image on screen. The difference between the two experiences taught me how to watch body gestures and not be distracted by what was being said. I also learned how to hear without being entranced by actions. This training helped me fine-tune my listening and observing skills, and enhanced the integration of my senses. I became responsive to others' needs and less focused on my own survival. The feedback I was able to give my patients aided them in bringing inner power to their vision.

I often ask my patients the question "How do you feel?" during a vision therapy session. As an exercise, ask yourself how *you* feel. Your feelings will be either switched on or switched off. If your feelings are switched off, then your response to the question might be "fine, good, okay, I don't know, neutral, plain, all right, average, so-so," even though you really might feel terrible. Switched-on feelings might produce responses such as "excited, thrilled, nervous, frustrated, sick, healthy, angry, full of fear, alive, like death, sad, grieving, uptight" to the same question.

Beginning to integrate your vision calls for telling the truth about how you really feel. Regardless of vision condition, my patients invariably need to learn how to express their feelings. I ask them to breathe below the throat by looking down and to the right when they speak. In this way, they maximize the possibility of accessing their feelings.

How do you feel? As you explore the answer, be in touch with yourself. Recall the differences between the fovea and retina. The retina has to do with feelings. If you are not in touch with your feelings, you are becoming too foveal. Too much *looking* is associated with being shut off from your feelings. Your focus on the details of life is too intense.

Contrast this with *being*, *seeing*, and *feeling*. These words mean being in touch with your soul. If you do not stay in touch with your feelings, you become detached from your retina. This is literally what happens, especially in higher degrees of nearsightedness. There is a higher probability of nearsighted people having retinal detachments. Is it possible that this occurs because of an overfocused fovea and a detachment from deeper fears and feelings? To feel is to consciously pay attention. To feel is to be mindful. Feeling requires exploring yourself. Be willing to take a moment to climb down from the attic of the mind, and enter the hearth and home of your soul-mind. Say: "Yes, my feelings are important. I count."

George

George was undecided about a career. He had started a small clothing business with a friend, which was bringing in some income. As I listened I heard that his real interests were music and photography. I asked George what he would most want to do if he had no restrictions of time, money, or fear. His answer: "I want to play music and do photojournalism." The heartfelt truth was out. The rest of the session was spent exploring how George was going to bring this vision into reality. This meant facing his fears. He had very skillfully learned how to hide his sensitivity and feelings. As I taught him to unify the left- and right-eye perceptions, using patching, eye-crossing, and fusion techniques, I encouraged him to share his feelings. George later reported that being in touch with his feelings was providing him with much more confidence in seeing his true self. This had a dramatic effect on his eyesight on the Far Eye-C chart.

Victim Vision

As much as I would like my patients to be as successful as George in enhancing their vision, sometimes the negative inner language and perceptions are too powerful, and they choose to see life through a filtering system of suffering. The "victim language" these patients use is quite typical: "I doubt." "I can't." "I'm not sure." Their behavior generally reveals a blaming attitude toward somebody or something outside of themselves. They lack ownership and responsibility for their reality and for the way they *see* life. The behavioral characteristics include being analytical, unforgiving, self-righteous, resigned, and in denial.

Julie

Julie, a patient in her mid-forties, consulted me because her physician had diagnosed her as having glaucoma, a potentially blinding condition. In glaucoma, constant pressure affects the backs of the eyes, which results in a blockage of the vital nerve supply to the eyes. This in turn creates greater pressure in the eye. Over time, glaucoma further and further reduces the field of vision.

Julie had used drops in her eyes for a short time, in order to keep the pressure down, but her work kept her so busy that she soon was forgetting to use the drops. "I love my work; it takes me out of the house," said Julie. She couldn't stand being alone. She was in denial of the relationship between the pressures of her life and the increased pressure in her eyes. Even after checking with an ophthalmologist, who warned that her visual fields were further reducing in size, Julie still did not fully embrace the Integrated Vision Therapy assignments I prescribed. I suggested she cut back her workload, hire other people, take a day off to get a massage, eat more wholesome foods, direct color into her eyes, and apply relaxation vision therapy.

I knew there were deeper reasons for the inner blindness that had been affecting her eyes. Julie was able to skillfully dodge my suggestions to feel. Instead, she talked in circles. Her favorite victim language was: "I don't know." I kept reminding her that she *did* know; she could *see* her truth, and I asked her to please *feel*. Many times Julie would turn the conversation around by asking me how I felt. When I was silent, she felt uncomfortable and accused me of staring at her.

I urged her to face the seriousness of the oncoming blindness that would result from the continuing loss of her peripheral visual field, but to no avail. She continued to take trips out of town, eat junk food, and repeat, "I don't know."

My role as Julie's vision therapist has been to encourage her to be receptive to the many variables that are responsible for the constriction in her eyes. To get herself to feel, she has been receiving massages once a week. A counseling component in her massage therapy has given Julie a chance to begin understanding the connection between her past and present family life and her eye condition.

Julie was sexually victimized as a young girl. Since that time, she has never been able to sleep in the dark. She must always keep a light on. She is very afraid. When she was nineteen, a man she was dating raped her. Julie became pregnant and gave birth to a daughter. These experiences set the stage for her avoidance of sexual intimacy with men.

Julie has not made love with her husband for many years. Even now, when her husband places his hand on her stomach, she freezes in fear and thinks she is going to be attacked. She describes her body as contracted, not unlike her constricted visual field. Her shoulders and stomach area are tight. A physician to whom I referred Julie diagnosed her as having a gluten allergy, which includes symptoms of poor digestion and emotional challenges.

Julie is making progress. She is now feeling more during her Integrated Vision Therapy activities. Occasionally she even cries. For a while the missing ingredient stalling Julie's progress was willingness to look deeply into her life. Julie's marriage was more codependent than it was truly supportive. Julie did not have real love in her life, and her job was too demanding. All these factors required her to take action to resolve past problems—to begin verbalizing her new perceptions and implement a plan for a new lifestyle. Julie had to learn to say what she wanted to see. It took a year of simply supporting her in this process, providing her with encouragement in the form of reminders, without any pressure. One day I received a phone call from Julie; she sounded desperate. Julie asked me to meet with her and her husband; he refused to believe that she wanted him to move out of the house. At last Julie took some action!

Julie is now living alone, getting ready to sell her house and business and begin a new life. The therapeutic foundation has been laid by Julie's willingness to verbalize her clear inner vision and put her plan into action, demonstrating her intention to disempower past influences. Julie continues to practice her vision games in order to restore balance in her nervous and visual systems and thus allow room for a loving relationship to come into her life. Julie has successfully begun dealing with the pressure in her life and how it has been affecting her eyes.

Tina

Tina was referred to me by friends whom I had also assisted. She limits her clarity by saying very little, and when she does speak, her language tends to suggest she is unaccountable. What she says confirms her mental approach to *seeing* life. This happens in spite of her excellent eyesight. Tina's challenge is to integrate her right- and left-eye perceptions in the presence of excellent eyesight. "I'm not sure" is Tina's favorite saying. Her body language communicates the same message. Her shoulders shrug. She often looks down, her head cocked to one side.

There is a vital link between this kind of head-tilt, astigmatism, and an interference in the integration of the perceptions from the two eyes. Take a moment to verify this for yourself. Play the vision game of eye uncrossing by placing your thumb between you and an object in front of you. Continue looking at the object until you can bring two thumbs into view. Now tilt your head, moving your right ear toward your right shoulder. Notice what happens to the height of the two thumbs. Angling your head into a slant can, in many cases, match the axis of the astigmatism. The greater the head tilt, the higher the probability that the two eyes are no longer able to integrate their respective images.

Tina didn't have astigmatism, but she had developed a competition between her Harry and Sally perceptions. Her right eye appeared visibly droopy and tired. Her language and facial asymmetry were that of a woman who was frustrated.

Tina worked for a large insurance company and had begun taking evening courses in Chinese medicine. At our first meeting, I asked her what she wanted. As she thought about the question her gaze wandered around the ceiling. This looking upward was a nonverbal representation of the language of the intellectual mind. Searching for the right verbal answer seemed to make Tina feel stuck. This impression was conveyed to me through the discomfort of her body posture.

Tina's way of working out her life was to constantly analyze and think about questions. I asked Tina to rub her hands together; the resulting friction warmed her palms. I then asked her to cover her eyes with her palms and place her elbows on her knees. This slight bending forward encouraged Tina to become more relaxed. I suggested she stay in this position for twenty integrated breaths, and coached her in relaxing her shoulders, neck, and mind. She began observing the blackness. I asked Tina to let out a sigh with each exhale. Making this sound required that Tina let go of her inhibitions and encouraged further relaxation.

Sounds can stimulate a person to feel certain fears. In this session with Tina, that is exactly what happened. Soon after palming, Tina shared more with me about her "stuck" life. She was afraid of not having enough money and had recently, at the age of twenty-eight, moved back in with her parents, who would take care of her. I expressed concern about this solution of "giving up" to her problems. After much questioning, Tina admitted that she disliked her job. She wanted to be independent and to help people. Her friends raved about her talents, but she lacked the confidence to take the plunge and reclaim her life. As Tina discovered the power behind her eyes, however, she became more able to *see* all the options available to her.

Becoming Empowered through Language

As you begin the journey of integrating your vision with your whole being, try to surround yourself with people who will be supportive of you. Begin to use language that supports what you want in your life. Develop the strength to communicate your needs. I have found these lead-in statements to be quite useful: "What will work for me, or what I need right now is . . . .

Will this work for you?" "My feelings are . . ." and "What I sense is . . ."

Use the following ideas to organize your thoughts and to adopt the concepts and activities from this chapter:

Write ten things you hear yourself say that you would like to modify.

Create ten positive statements that you can begin using immediately.

Do you use victim language? If so, begin using more positive language.

Use the Far or Near Eye-C chart to experience the effect of using your negative and positive statements. Are you aware of feelings while looking at the charts? Go deeper into your feelings by breathing and yawning.

During your day, continue to check in with yourself by saying, "How I feel right now is . . ."

As feelings emerge, focus your attention on your heart area. Begin to feel and see from the heart. What does your heart have to say to you? Examine your career, your personal relationships, and your home life to see if you can honestly say: "This is what I want." If not, in what other direction are you guided to look from an integrated point of view? What new avenues do you wish to explore?

Looking at yourself in a holistic way, what aspects of yourself do you wish to give more consideration? Can you clearly verbalize these thoughts to bring them into action? The act of imaging these thoughts, then talking or writing about them, enables you to project your new clarity outside of yourself.

Complete this statement in several different ways: "What I really want is . . ." Complete the sentence as many times as necessary, until you become clear.

Are there situations in your life where you could tape-record yourself speaking? Do so, and listen to yourself for variations in your voice that reveal you are giving your power away. Does your voice remind you of a particular family member? If so, what feelings do you have? Write them down.

Do you play the victim in any areas of your life? If so, list them on paper and produce action statements to defuse these behaviors.

Try to remember issues or events in your life that may be related to your vision being the way it is.

Choose two new forms of relaxation that you can use to improve your vision and clarity.

Where in your life do you diminish your power to *see*? Pay attention to when you use the disempowering language from the column on the left and learn to start replacing it with the empowering language from the column on the right:

I don't know	I know, I see
I hope	I am clear
I can't	I am
I doubt	I am looking at
Maybe	Yes! I will
I'll try	You can count on me
It's OK	My experience is
I'm fine	I feel
Possibly	I am sure
I'm not sure	My intention is
I suppose	I am clear that
I forget	I remember
I'll get back to you	You will hear from me by

Jenny

Jenny, a warm woman in her mid-forties, was committed to balancing her personality with her soul. Her goal was to maintain her vision and to prevent it from getting worse. At –15.00, her nearsightedness was severe enough that her ophthalmologist was concerned about the health of the retina, future detachments, and loss of eyesight. Jenny took the initiative to learn Integrated Vision Therapy techniques to safeguard her eyes. Even though the forecast for improved vision was slim, Jenny moved quickly from a position of despair to one of anticipation. She stated, "I will do anything to help prevent my eyes from getting worse." A strong statement of action. I knew that with this kind of willingness, I had total permission to guide her in the choices necessary to reach her goal.

Relaxation was a key for Jenny. Palming her eyes and massaging the eyebrow area with her index fingers produced relaxation around her eyes. This reduced the tendency for Jenny to frown and also helped her to think less and feel more. Feeling her body sensations was a critically important step. Her job forced her to look at a computer screen eight hours a day. Jenny's eyes ached by the end of the day. When she experienced a decline in her eyesight, she became depressed and began to hate her job, although she loved the contact with people. Jenny had faced challenges with money and had moved back in with her father because she was overextended. Jenny's first emotional feelings about her situation came out in the form of anger.

The most effective vision therapy technique for dealing with anger is stretching the jaw muscles. Practice yawning. Open your mouth as wide as you can and take a couple of small in-breaths as you do. This will help you spontaneously yawn. Repeat until your eyes begin to water. You may feel tension in the jaw muscles at first, but soon they will relax. This release of muscle tension facilitates letting go of anger, according to Australian physician John Harrison. In his book entitled *Love Your Disease; It's Keeping You Healthy,* Dr. Harrison maintains that the physiological responses of a wide pupil (an indication of an overactive sympathetic nervous system), high adrenaline levels, and elevated blood pressure are related to the presence of anger in the muscles. As the anger is dealt with, these physiological measurements return to normal levels. The distressing challenge occurs when you bury the anger.

Soon after she began Integrated Vision Therapy, Jenny was better able to see how to organize her finances. She moved out of her father's house and began investing in rental-income properties. Her goal was to have a secure income for her retirement years. These ventures still kept her "in her head," and as she was slightly overweight, I suggested she begin gardening. Working in the soil gave Jenny the chance to leave her mental mind and to feel her body. Gardening helped bring her out of the thinking into the feeling part of her being.

The real challenge for Jenny, who thrived on getting information from books, came when I suggested that she not read for three months. This directive might sound quite severe, but Jenny needed to stop putting her eyes and vision under so much strain. Reading is unnatural for the eyes. The eyes are designed for looking off into the distance and for short periods of close focusing. Reading activates the mental part of the brain. Since Jenny spent so much time at the computer, I also designed a special computer-based vision therapy maintenance program for her. This included eye uncrossing, shifting her focus around the screen, palming, and monitoring her vision fitness on the Far Eye-C chart. Jenny also took more rest breaks to keep her vision clear during the day.

Jenny's eyesight varied, and therefore her contact lenses were often uncomfortable. I did not pressure her to give up contacts in preference to eyeglasses. Since she had made a twelve-month commitment to her vision therapy process, I waited. I knew that as her vision stabilized she would one day be unable to wear her strong contact lenses. Jenny came in one day six months after we'd begun working together and told me that she had not worn her contact lenses for three weeks. She reverted to her old eyeglasses, which she had previously worn only at night. Her former red and overstrained eyes seemed more relaxed, and she proudly told me that she had ordered weaker eyeglasses.

Jenny recently chose to have laser surgery, which according to her has been very successful in reducing her need to wear contacts or strong glasses. Jenny acknowledged the value of Integrated Vision Therapy in preparing her for her new vision. I photographed her eyes prior to the surgery and will be closely following her progress. On the surface Jenny is happy. She has resolved her eyesight difficulty, and superficially appears not to consider herself a victim. I am of the opinion that Jenny's personality- or ego-driven state has still not fully integrated with her intuitive being, resulting in the holding back of her full soul presence. Jenny came a long way with her Integrated Vision Therapy and then chose to abort. When Jenny is ready to merge her ego, intuition, and soul, then she will fully experience the power and sacred nature of multidimensional vision.

Chapter 7

Your Secret Purpose

Why Are You Here?

Dr. Dean Ornish says his spiritual teacher, Swami Satchitananda, frequently asked him: "What is the cause?" The swami was referring to the cause of the degenerating heart conditions of Dr. Ornish's patients. Upon receiving a superficial answer, the teacher kept asking, "Yes, but what is the cause? And what is the cause of that? And what underlies that cause?" These questions helped Dr. Ornish design a progressive program for reversing heart disease based on a very relevant premise: Address the underlying causes, which is ultimately more effective than addressing only the symptoms.

So when you state, as do many of my patients, that you wish to improve your vision, I ask, "When you have accomplished this, then what? Why are you here? What is your life for?" Are you here to only pay mortgages, shop in malls, and read the bad news in magazines and newspapers? Do these activities inspire you and contribute to your well-being?

Once you have faced your symptoms of blurry and distorted vision due to errors of refraction and disease in your eyes, then what? Pretend for a moment that you are given another opportunity to live. If you had no restrictions, how would you spend your day? Examine what you have created. Sometimes my patients don't change their lives; they develop a deeper appreciation for what they already have. Others make major life changes. Sybil, a patient in her forties, improved her eyesight and, in the process, gave up nursing others. She realized that finally she needed to nurse herself.

Living is awakening your soul. If indeed we do reincarnate, then how do our activities enhance or take away from our souls? Are you like many others who are selling their soul for the next paycheck? In their book *Your Money or Your Life,* authors Joe Dominguez and Vicki Robin propose that we *could* be living a life of passion, serving humankind with worthwhile projects and being financially well-rewarded for our time. Simple needs with clear resolution will help you find your niche.

What is your heartfelt contribution? What stimulates your self-worth? Find your mission. Create a plan. Choose a quiet moment and write down your vision for your life. Verbalize your insights by talking to a close friend. Then spend time on activities that inspire you to be in accord with your nature. Inspiration will follow. Peace of mind sets in. You feel more healthy and alive. Your eyes will heal and your vision will sharpen.

The essence of achieving good vision is the readiness to see yourself as you really are—a kind and good person. In my own case, I participated in personal development programs in which I received feedback about how others perceived me as wise. At first, the meaning of wisdom was a foreign concept to me. As I looked inside and honestly assessed how I saw myself, I felt incompetent, lazy, and a failure. My academic accomplishments were based on my survival-based instincts and the domination of my personality. By accepting the wisdom others saw in me, I noticed my vision improving. I practiced focusing my intention on the primal goodness that was present within me. This daily practice of stillness increased my awareness of my wisdom and my soul. I consciously began to take time out from my *doing* lifestyle to notice the beauty of my surroundings. I took better care of myself. I saw more of my own goodness, which translated into seeing the goodness in everything around me.

Although much of the New Age movement attempts to teach this goodness, goodness cannot be accessed mentally, as a concept. However, in these modern times, people think they can "get it" in a weekend seminar. Unless goodness is rooted in your daily life, your visual transformation will be elusive and transient. This is partly why vision therapy has taken so long to catch on. People viewed this transforming therapy as fixing something wrong with the *eyes*—learn a few exercises and they will repair the problem. To be good and to *see* clearly requires accessing your core essence and identifying your real motives.

Probably there are events in your life that have set in motion a visual inflexibility. You may tend to limit yourself in your visual options. Consider one or two of the visually related events you have uncovered so far. In retrospect, what can you learn from these circumstances? At each stage, as your vision unfolds, new understanding can emerge as you realize the good that has emerged. Review past situations to uncover new insights about them and your automatic reactions to them.

Flexibility is the openness to interpret the events that occur in life from many points of view. During our childhood most perceptual decisions are influenced by our relationships with our parents or teachers. At a younger age we may reflexively behave in a "doing it right" manner. We want to be clear but we may still behave in order to please. During these times our behavior can be more reactive than responding. When we look from a re- actionary posture, we tend to see only one solution in the instant of react- ing. To be responsive means to see from stillness and to see that the situation is a good one, no matter how challenging it may seem. Many points of view and options exist.

Our reactions to life's experiences actually limit the ability of our eyes to receive and transmit light. This physical inadequacy creates mispercep- tions in the way we observe life. Our first knee-jerk reactions to an event are based on the misperceptions we carry with us. These automatic re- sponses cause us to perceive things in a predetermined, habitual way.

Being aware of the clarity or blurring of your vision gives you the op- portunity to open up new synaptic and perceptual pathways in your brain. Physical changes such as reducing near- or farsightedness, reducing astig- matism, reducing the pressure inside your eye, healing retinal tissue, mini- mizing floaters, and sharpening your eyesight can actually take place. Visual flexibility is possible when you become aware of how you are seeing events in your life.

Clarity is accurate perceiving by looking through your heart. The goal is to perceive your own life through your eyes and your heart, rather than through the veil of your genetic perceptions as translated through your logi- cal mind. Seeing through this veil is like seeing your life through someone else's eyes. When you lift the veil of your present misperceptions, you be- gin to trust yourself, and your life takes on new meaning. You will begin to trust the way you see your life and the others in it.

Recall the vertical and horizontal aspects of vision that I discussed in chapter 1 while describing astigmatism. As a way of accessing your verti- cal energy flow, imagine that a cord of energy links the sky to the earth, uniting you with the power centers in the sky, giving you the ability to feel the power and beauty of life flow effortlessly through you. Through this intangible connection, life feels like less of a struggle. Practice sensing that flow of energy moving through you as you breathe. Feel the energy surge inside you, entering up through your anus and traveling through your body to the top of your head. (Even though you may think that nothing is happening at first, this exercise creates a flow of energy through your power centers, the chakras.) The more you can allow this energy to move through you, the more power you have to bring forth your secret purpose.

Many psychotherapies involve focusing on the past. While it is important to identify deep-seated core issues and deal with them, the past is but one place to focus; it is only a reflection. You must live your life in the here and now. You would not drive your car while looking out the back window to see where you have been. Instead, from the driver's seat, you look into the journey ahead, knowing you can draw on your past experiences if you need to.

The world is not here to judge you or to validate who you are. You are capable of validating your own perceptions and of determining the reality of what you see today. When you choose a new perceptual path in life, no matter how much of a challenge it may appear to be, stay committed to being on that path until you reach your goals. If you begin to doubt your new perceptions, simply stop and sharpen your awareness by looking at your life clearly, without fear. When you race through life, you speed past things you are afraid of. "I am not used to spending so much time on myself," said one of my patients in the course of her home vision therapy. When you slow down, you are able to *see* your truth and what you really want.

Start becoming aware of times when your perceptions are aligned with your truth, when you feel right and comfortable with yourself. What body sensations do you feel when your life is going well and you are seeing clearly? Observe the issues from the past that surface during your Integrated Vision Therapy practice. How can you deal with that past issue from your current higher level of awareness? Imagine yourself completing the need to dwell on that issue and *see* a fresh vision for the situation. See this new idea flourishing, and let your eyes receive this clear programming.

Life transformation comes about through daily focus and practice. Vision enhancement is similar. Seeing clearly and being focused means discovering your secret purpose for living. Your purpose is the frame into which you place the picture of the life you wish to create.

For now, it will be useful for you to start exploring ways of identifying or rediscovering your purpose. I use the word *rediscovering* because somewhere along the path of life, most of us lose touch with the simple, honest clarity and focus we enjoyed as children—a time when we thought we could be anything we wanted to be when we grew up. As your clear vision of life reemerges, your eyes will experience healthier vision. When you remove, overcome, or set aside fears and obstructions that restrict you from really living your truth, your innate goodness begins to shine through.

As you contemplate unfinished aspects of your life that contribute to losing your eyesight, keep in mind that you cannot "fix" the past, but you *can* remove the veils of the past that have been hiding your purpose for existing.

The Tibetan Dür Bön tradition teaches that your soul enters your physical body sometime during the first three months in utero. A soul chooses a physical body to complete "unfinished business." No matter what you initially *think* your life is about, your soul has a deeper purpose.

To have *vision* is to see your soul's purpose for existing. It is easy to concentrate on the physical and tangible aspects of living, and you can be easily seduced into believing that your physical body is the most important aspect of life. Many of my patients begin their vision journey believing that their only intent is to repair the problem they are having with their eyes. Sooner or later, however, they are confronted with the emptiness of their physical lives. What they see through their vision no longer matches their perceptions from the past. They start to ask questions such as "What is my real purpose for being here?" "What plan does my soul have for me?" "What will be the consequence if I do not pay attention to my soul's needs?" I once saw a bumper sticker that read: My Karma ran over your Dogma. All we can do is drive our own karma, taking responsibility for and then seeing the bigger picture of our lives.

A patient recently told me how much she had learned from her eyes. When she was very young Angel's right eye turned inward. She had undergone two surgical procedures on her right eye, and when that didn't work her ophthalmologist sliced into the muscles of her left eye to resolve the problem. The surgery was intended to alter the muscle length so that the eye would align itself. The procedures had left her with massive scar tissue on both eyes.

For years afterward, she experienced pain in her eyes and episodes of blurry vision; the agony forced her to face tremendous lessons in her life and to ask the deeper question, "What is my purpose on this planet?" She found she had to explore her past in order to better define her current healing strategy.

Abe and Sophie fell in love and realized they wanted to spend their lives together. They married and decided to travel around the world for a year and then settle down to have a family.

The Story of Abe and Sophie

While Abe and Sophie are on holiday, their son Alex, still in the spiritual realm, decides to arrive on his own schedule. Alex senses that the timing for coming to earth is perfect. A while later, he makes his appearance inside of Sophie.

Alex thinks, "What a perfect time to be developing. I am sharing all this rest and relaxation time, and my parents are so loving and caring toward each other. There is hardly any stress. We swim in the gorgeous blue-green waters of Greece, Fiji, South Africa, and Australia. The food they are eating is healthy, and my parents are getting plenty of exercise. What a time to choose to be in utero. I feel pampered and respected as a new being on this planet."

After eight months, Abe and Sophie return home. Alex is getting big inside the womb. His parents are planning a water birth at home. Alex is content. "My parents are so progressive. That is why I chose them. What they don't realize is that I wanted the underwater birth. After all, I am a Scorpio; I love water. They think they are going to be my parents. This is true but I have something in store for them. My soul is powerful and I am preparing them for the greatest teaching they have ever had." Your own personality was molded when you were in utero. Your parents' state of *being* at the time you were conceived, while you were in utero, during your birth, and in your early years, impacted the way you *see* life.

Your soul purpose, your reason for being, may have been dampened by the attitudes and beliefs transmitted by your parents' conscious and unconscious actions. But each event that resulted in the soul's being suppressed later becomes an opportunity for you to grow. The people with the greatest hardships in many cases turn out to contribute the greatest to life. If your parents are alive, ask them to give you an emotional account of your conception, birth, and early years. Were they happy? Where were they in their journey of unfolding consciousness? Can they remember difficult times in your life that you may be able to chronologically link to your eye problems? Add this information to your other discoveries so far. Tennyson's Ulysses says: "I am a part of all that I have met." Every event from your past has made you who you are today. Honor your past and be who you are! The more you know about your past, the greater clarity you can bring into the present and future.

If you are contemplating having children, pregnancy is a chance for you to grow personally. Take time out from work, and speak to the little one inside you. The movement of your body, the sound of your voice, and the vital nutrients from the wholesome foods you consume will nurture your child's future awakening of purpose.

Simon

At age fourteen, Simon had only one real desire: to become a helicopter pilot in the army. But his eyes were measured as nearsighted. This perceptual constriction was caused by Simon's feeling that he had to fulfill some role his parents or teachers desired for him. Simon's developing personality was living a life that was untrue to his soul's itinerary. His father brought him to see me out of guilt for not spending enough time with him. He had a great wish to help his son *see* and lead his life with more purpose than before.

Of the three children in the family, Simon was the only one who wore glasses, and he needed a stronger prescription each year. He did not wear his glasses unless he wanted to see the board at school. Watching his face and eyes, I saw a lot of tension and "trying-to-see" behavior. His left eye perceived more clearly and was more dominant, and he also favored his left-eyed perception while playing the two-thumb game. This meant he was very perceptive, and he needed to further develop this sensitivity. He was an excellent musician, played rugby, and enjoyed fishing. I taught him how to palm his eyes, stimulate the face and brow muscles, breathe from the heart, and activate acupressure points with his fingers. Then I told him this story:

A teenager very much wanted to fly an airplane, but he had been told his vision would never be good enough to make him eligible. His father heard of an eye doctor who taught his patients to see clearer with less dependency on eyeglasses. He visited this doctor for a couple of hours, and every day for the next twelve months he faithfully did all the vision exercises he had been taught. He was passionate about seeing better. He visualized himself flying F-16 jets. Today, this man is flying jets. I told Simon that I was that boy's eye doctor.

Simon was visibly moved. His face seemed to relax, and I encouraged him to open his eyes wider. I then proceeded to give him and his father further homework. Simon was to take up painting nature scenes to stimulate his discernment of vision as an artistic endeavor rather than a mental one. He was to patch his right eye as he painted outside. Also, he was to volunteer to be around older people. When Simon talked to them, he would experience his own wisdom through being with them.

Craig

Following his parents' expectations, Craig had teamed up with his father to manage the family sheep and cattle farm, the same farm he grew up on. Craig described his life as being entrenched, and he couldn't see a way out. He hung onto wearing his eyeglasses in the same needy way. (Neither parent wore glasses, so his nearsightedness and astigmatism were not genetically coded in the family tree.)

Craig's left eye had significantly more astigmatism to the point where he didn't fully integrate the two perceptions through each eye. For thirty-eight years, Craig had disciplined his vision to *look* through the right eye—a Harry-dominated view of the world. He would look at life through his logical filtering system, carefully masking any feelings. His inner knowing about the emotional and soul side of his mind was latent.

Craig answered every question with "I don't know." He had had only brief relationships with women, and he used a slight hearing loss and a fear of traveling as excuses for not leaving the farm. His behavior suggested a keen interest in improving his vision, but he felt stuck.

Vision exercises alone were not going to move this man. Craig needed a bomb underneath him to achieve the kind of changes he desired for himself. We began a patching program for his right eye. As he performed his farming duties wearing the patch, he was developing a left-eye perception of the world.

As is the case in most patching exercises, Craig had to slow down and pay more attention to his world through his left (Sally-perceiving) eye. He had to feel what he was seeing, rather than only thinking about it. He learned to transfer this new way of observing to his other assignments.

When sitting quietly, Craig used the eye crossing and uncrossing vision game (see chapter 3). While looking at his thumb in front of his eyes, Craig began to follow the thumb with his eyes, moving along the exact blurry meridian of his astigmatism (in this case, along the horizontal). This stimulated the blocked nerve pathway from his brain to his eye. Next, he had to face some lifestyle changes. Craig had never cooked for himself nor attempted to set up house. His mother had always taken care of him. He wanted to have a relationship with a woman but couldn't see clearly enough through the left-eye side of his perceptual consciousness to make this a reality.

I suggested he move away from his parents' farm and take an apartment in the nearby town. In addition, he was to take a six-month sabbatical from farming. Living in the town and preparing for his holiday, Craig would face his fears, step out of his comfort zone, and take a risk. His nearsightedness and astigmatism represented living in a nonrisking realm. Integrating his vision through this therapy meant reaching out to the unknown. Being in town and patching his right eye would give Craig the chance to make new friends and begin the journey of reaching for his own dreams and personal vision.

Pauleen

Craig's sister Pauleen also came to visit me. She had excellent eyesight but had difficulty seeing the two candles or thumbs when she uncrossed her eyes. Her dominant perception was through her left eye.

Pauleen was a loving woman who, like Craig, had spent a secluded early life on the farm. When she did leave she fell in and out of relationships. She stated that her mother had never shared her deepest feelings, and Pauleen missed having an emotional connection with her mother and brother. Her nature was emotional and loving, but she had no role model for creating close relationships. As a young girl she swore that when she had children, they would talk a lot about their feelings.

While living away from the farm, Pauleen met a suitable man. They had a short and intense relationship, and she was devastated when he suddenly left her for another woman. Pauleen retreated once more to the farm. Her ability to integrate her two-eyed perceptions became worse, and she lived in fear of being abandoned by men. Not much later, she met the man who was to be her husband. Within a month, they announced their engagement and married. Two children were born to them.

Even though it looked as though Pauleen had plenty of security, her perceptions of life were tainted by her inner perceptions of fear. Each time her husband left for a trip, she panicked, thinking he might not return. How would she manage if her fear of abandonment came true? On deeper questioning, she admitted that she harbored resentment toward her brother and her family.

Pauleen was ready to begin the integration process and to claim her right to her power. This meant patching her eye and facing her brother and her family in a loving and compassionate way. To prepare Pauleen for this endeavor, I suggested she begin developing a closer relationship with a particular female friend. They were to meet for two hours each week, at which time they would give each other a massage and talk about personal matters. This was important for Pauleen, because her husband was the only person she ever talked to on an intimate level. He was a great listener and would freely give her advice. This pattern of relying on her husband as her only intimate contact added to Pauleen's sense that she was dependent on her husband for everything.

Through her right eye, Pauleen began to develop strength of perception. She became more independent. As she applied this freedom, her power returned. Her vision became more multidimensional. While fusing objects, she could maintain her integrated state and ask for what she wanted. This also transformed her relationship with her parents, siblings, and friends.

Childhood Dreams

Identify situations in your own life in which you gave away your power to someone else's vision of what was best for you. You can recapture your soul purpose. The initial step is to assess your life with your parents or caregivers. What dilemmas in their lives influenced your early decisions? After asking the question, consider how you might regain this power and use it productively in your life. If your vision problem developed during later years, think about how that might relate to the people who were the closest to you at the time. When you stimulate your memory of the past, you can better understand how your way of perceiving things was shaped, and how it has molded the way you have been living your life.

In an effort to remember the early influences that shaped your life, ask yourself the following questions and write your responses.

> What do you know about your birth experience (cesarean, long labor, breech birth, etc.)?
>
> Did your parents ever separate or divorce? If so, how do you feel about those events now?
>
> Were you born out of wedlock?
>
> Did your parents have any addictive behaviors, such as smoking, drinking, or overworking?
>
> Did your family move to a new home more than once during your early years?
>
> Did any of your family members exhibit habitually angry or loud behavior?
>
> When you were a child, did a significant friend move away? Did you and your family move away from your significant friend?
>
> Where you physically, sexually, or emotionally abused?
>
> Can you recall having to deal with death early in life?
>
> Did your parents have problems with lack of money and financial security?
>
> Where there any negative situations in your schooling that stand out?
>
> Can you recall your first visit to an eye doctor?
>
> Did the eye doctor say anything that may have influenced your vision or your decisions about seeing? (He could have said it to your parents, in your company.)
>
> Have you ever used reading as an escape mechanism?
>
> Did you read in poor light as a child?
>
> Did your parents wear glasses? Did this have any influence on your vision? (Did you want to wear glasses because your mom or dad wore them?)
>
> Were there periods in your life when you ate excessive amounts of sugar, dairy products, or meat products?

Having looked back into your past, now see into the future. Consider these questions. Your responses will help you see your tomorrow more clearly.

Do you want to improve your vision to please someone else?

Do you expect to be changing your career as you become clearer in your perceptions?

By accessing the power behind your eyes, will you be earning more money?

Do you think you will move from your present home within the next twelve months?

Do you anticipate beginning a new relationship within the next year?

If you wear glasses, can you visualize yourself wearing progressively weaker lens prescriptions?

If you have an eye disease, can you imagine going back to your eye doctor and receiving the good news that your eye tissue is becoming healthy?

Do you see yourself spending time contributing one of your skills or services to your community?

When you were very young, your dreams were the initial expression of your soul manifesting itself in the world. I am not referring only to the pictures that surfaced while you were sleeping. Dreams occur while you are awake, during your play and your creative pursuits. These are the insights that help produce the essence of who you are.

I remember being a nonreader as a child, and yet I was fascinated by books on psychology. I would spend hours in our town library scanning psychology books in an attempt to understand my family's behavior and my own. In addition to this fascination with psychology, I took up photography, partly because it was also my father's interest. Yet deep within my own core, photography was my artistic form of expression, and I found I needed that outlet for expressing my emotions. As a Boy Scout, I also enjoyed the outdoors and being self-sufficient.

When I look back at my childhood pursuits, I realize the intense effect my early education had on creating an imbalance between my personality and my soul. I was encouraged to focus upon academics, and I believed that this is where I should excel; yet, because of my double vision and my need to over-focus, I lost touch with some of my intuitive abilities. I have subsequently acknowledged that my soul is calling me to lead a simple life of being a supportive husband, raising my children, and teaching and helping others.

Give yourself an opportunity to explore your childhood dreams. Ask yourself the following questions and write your responses.

Name five things you were clear about before you were ten years old.

How many of these early dreams have you implemented into your current daily living?

Are any of these dreams still important in your life? If so, what do you
need to do to make them happen?

What are your current dreams or visions for yourself? How can you include these in your work, personal life, or recreational activities?

If you are a parent, encourage your child to talk to you about his or
her dreams. Ask your child to fantasize about their future. Support the
sharing of these insights at the dinner table with the family, or before the
child goes to sleep. One prime way you can stimulate your child's visualizing mode is to limit the amount of television he or she watches. In his book
Evolution's End, Joseph Chilton Pearce argues ardently that creativity in
children can be hindered by their watching television. Psychological literature abounds with provocative research on how children's behavior is modified by excessive television viewing.

At age two, our son Symon became engrossed with watching children's
videos; he loved to view the images on the screen. During those times, my
wife and I enjoyed the opportunity to have quiet time and a break from
parenting. However, we were horrified at Symon's angry behavior every time
we suggested that it was time to turn off the video. We became aware that
Symon was addicted to the television. We began setting a timer for ten-minute
viewing periods. This started a weaning process that took a few months.

In the meantime, we began taping the video material onto audio-
cassettes. This meant we could switch off the television monitor and let
him listen to his videos. This was hilarious to watch. Symon still glared at
the video screen while he listened. I am sure he was seeing the image projected from his mind onto the screen. Within a few weeks he began playing with his toys while he listened—he was seeing the images in his mind.

If you wish to help your child maintain the power behind his or her
eyes, include positive statements just prior to the child's dozing off to sleep.
For my son, I create a story. While lying down with him at night, I start off
by saying, "Symon is lovable and huggable. Symon is cooperative and beautiful. Symon is a bright light. Symon is intelligent and healthy. Symon is
generous and capable. Symon is loved by his mother and father. Symon is
spiritual and a teacher. Symon is helpful and understanding," and so on.
While he passes into the early stages of sleep, these statements are being
absorbed and stored in his brain.

The next stage is to have your child begin verbalizing positive statements him- or herself. I have found that these suggestions help neutralize
the negative behavior inherited from the genealogical past. As these per-

sonality aspects reveal themselves, the soul is balanced by these gentle caring words. Up to the age of seven, your child's capacity to integrate these compassionate feelings is wide open, even during waking hours.

I remember a client who was having behavioral problems with her six-year-old daughter. Barbara was a single mother whose boyfriend had recently moved in with her. Pam, her daughter, was a handful. Everything Barbara said produced a negative reaction from Pam. Pam's antagonistic and willful behavior was causing a breakdown in Barbara's communication with her boyfriend and making it difficult for them even to live together. Pam's first-grade teacher commented to Barbara that Pam was finding it difficult to get along with her school friends.

Barbara and Pam

As Barbara was one of my Integrated Vision Therapy patients, I suggested I meet Pam to see if I could be of assistance in the situation. The visit was most challenging. Pam would not sit still and kept shoving her mother away. Most of the time, she sat curled up on the couch and would not respond to my playful interactions. I managed to entice her into sitting still so that I could take photographs of her iris patterns.

Pam's eyes and her mother's eyes were distinctly different. The source of Pam's agitation was that she was negatively expressing genealogical traits from her father's side of the family. Using the Rayid method of iris interpretation described earlier, I looked at Pam's right-eye photograph and was able to determine that Pam had a very emotional nature. She needed activities that would allow her to express this emotion in a positive way.

Each time she returned from a visit with her father, Pam needed three days to calm down. After reading her iris, I was able to create a number of reinforcing statements that Barbara read into a tape recorder. At night, while putting Pam to sleep, she played the tape. She also enrolled Pam in an art class so she could express her personality through positive, guided creativity.

Within a few weeks, the dividends of this form of therapy paid off. Pam's teacher was amazed at the changes in Pam's behavior. Pam's personality seemed more balanced, and she began to reveal the loving and caring side of her nature. Listening to the tape helped neutralize Pam's negative emotions. Barbara was reminded of the need for her own essential healing, which included speaking in a more direct manner to her ex-husband. Shortly thereafter, Barbara's eyesight through weaker contact lenses, prescribed as part of her vision therapy, began to sharpen when she checked herself on the Far Eye-C chart.

The Light Within

The light that enters our eyes is coded by a primitive organ in the brain called the pineal gland, to stimulate the brain's consciousness of perceptions. Color from light also colors your essence and awakens your soul. The Buddhists believe that when light primes your body's metabolism, the root cause of unclear vision becomes apparent. Your body remembers how to see.

Most of us had clear eyesight at birth, and then it dimmed. While you were becoming acculturated, blurring of your inherent goodness set in. The Flowering Light Tantra from the Tibetan Dür Bön tradition states: "Your body is your memory in form. Your body has something to reveal. Your eyes are endeavoring to apprise you of your essential heart." Your vision from your heart gives the eyes a portal from which to look through. Your eyes only respond to what you perceive to be true. When you look from the heart, you will be able to clearly see your undiscovered purpose.

Your outward vision emerges from a still mind. The Talmud advises, "You can only see what the mind projects." It takes stillness to really see through your eyes. When you are relaxed, your mind has an increased capacity to perform miraculous tasks.

The light within is stimulated in great part when you relax, allow sunlight to enter your eyes, and feel a deep connection with nature. As you develop skill at the practice of integrated breathing with your eyes open, you will feel more in tune with the cycles of nature around you. Wake up early one morning and practice integrated breathing outside, while the sun is rising. My favorite summer activity is to go to the beach, sit quietly, and let the early morning sun bathe my face.

Listen. There are a multitude of sounds in the early morning. Each living species has a language and communication of its own. As you open your eyes to these life forms, you will become aware of their distinctive radiating light. Since light is energy, all living matter emanates light. You do too. Your eyes receive and convey light. When your emotional reactions dominate and you lose touch with life, especially with the visual beauty of nature, the capacity of your eyes to receive light diminishes.

If you have difficulty seeing the printed page as light levels drop, perhaps your message is to stop reading. Experiment with restricting your reading to daylight hours. In small ten-minute exposures early in the morning or just prior to sunset, let light from the sun wake up your inner calmness. Move your head back and forth and blink often. Of course, avoid looking directly at the sun. As you become accustomed to letting the light of the sun in, you will find your power returning. If you are allergic to bright sunlight, your Harry or Sally perceptions are not integrating at the highest possible level. Alternatively, you may have overtaxed your liver by eating foods too rich in oils or fats. The more you relax and integrate your two-eyed vision, the more you will be able to receive light.

Your brainwaves, measured on an electroencephalogram, look like ocean waves. The most well-known of the brainwaves is the alpha state. This level of brain function produces artistic or mindful levels of perception. Hypnosis, meditation, integrated breathing, and induced states of relaxation are practices that produce alpha rhythms in the brain. If you continually remain in a thinking, intellectual mode, you are less able to relax into alpha. Many people are stuck in their heads and are not able to relax their bodies.

One of my patients, a thirty-year-old woman, underwent hypnotic age-regression that took her back to age nineteen, when her first glasses were prescribed. She relaxed so much during the hypnosis that when she opened her eyes, she was effectively at that younger age in her mind. Her eyesight was measured at age thirty. When she regressed to the age of eighteen (a time before she wore glasses), her eyesight was again assessed. A significant degree of blur was present when she was thirty, whereas her eyesight at age eighteen was a perfect 20/20. I have witnessed similar improvements in eyesight just by having my patients relax through integrated breathing while they wear weaker lens prescriptions. When you practice the integrated breathing while watching a candle or being in nature, deepen your relaxation. Know that you too can go back in time and see clearly. Each reduction in lens prescription that you make is bringing you closer to your dreams and purpose. Go back in time and discover the clearness of vision that a part of you can still remember. You are awakening your deepest perceptions, so keep a written record and be prepared to face whatever emerges on your journey.

The first step toward accomplishing inner focus is to eliminate all extraneous clutter from your life and complete all those things that are now half-finished. Inventory the places where you work and live. List in a journal the things that distract you from being with yourself: these might include a job in which you feel unfulfilled; old furniture that no longer suits you; closets full of clothes you don't wear; incomplete legal or accounting matters, or correspondence; mechanical items in poor repair; partners, lovers, friends, or roommates who seem to drain your energy; incomplete communication with friends or family; a car that costs more to maintain than it's worth; ignored hobbies, books, and other items you haven't looked at for more than a year; broken promises; unpaid debts; and so forth. After completing your list, consider how these items have the power to influence your capacity to be still, to be inside yourself and to focus on your real needs. Plan to begin cleaning out those things that no longer serve you and your life purpose.

Spend a week changing your normal pattern of doing things. Get out of bed from the other side or change the side you usually sleep on. If you watch TV at night, leave it off. If you read at night, choose another activity, or simply sit still in quietness. Rather than spending twenty minutes to prepare and eat a meal, give yourself an hour and a half, and savor the experience. Take a bath instead of showering. Remove your contacts or leave your eyeglasses off in the evening at home. Begin to vary your life conditions to awaken other parts of your perceptual consciousness. When you are in your blur, and you change your habitual conditioning, you rely more on your inner focus, and this awakens your soul. Write about your experiences in your journal.

I assist my patients to identify their preferred eye by sighting through a paper tube, as if looking through a telescope. You can perform this experiment yourself. Using a tube or a rolled piece of paper and holding it with both hands, note which eye you automatically choose to look through. This is your preferred-sighting eye. Now select an object to look at, either with or without your eyeglasses. Cover one eye with the palm of your hand, then cover the other eye. Notice if one of your eyes sees more clearly than the other. While you are relaxing at home, cover your preferred eye with a patch. Everything will seem to slow down around you. It will feel to you as if half of you has disappeared. Experience the loss of depth perception you feel when you attempt to pick up an object. Begin experimenting with the patch while performing a variety of safe activities, such as balancing a checkbook, writing, cooking, cleaning, and ironing.

Patching one eye demands that the part of the brain associated with the other eye wake up and *see*. Recall that each eye has its own perceptual character. Looking through the right eye evokes perceptual qualities associated with analysis, logic, and detailed focus, while looking through the left eye evokes feelings, emotions, and creativity. This patching activity asks the brain to focus in a different way than in our usual way of perceiving when both eyes are open. Build up to longer and longer periods of wearing the patch on one eye, up to a maximum of four hours a day if possible. The purpose of looking through one eye at a time is to explore your perceptions and program your new awareness of the experience into the brain.

After you remove the patch, the intensity of light will seem much greater, and you will feel a different sense of integration—that of seeing through both eyes. Your focus will be broader. Colors will seem brighter. Through the patching technique, you'll understand how you focus through your eyes.

The feeling of slowing down when one eye is covered gives us the opportunity to tune inward. We are undoing our normal ways of perceiving and opening up new possibilities of seeing in the mind. It is very seductive to stay too busy, looking outside of ourselves for the answers to life's many challenges. We escape to television, books, and computers to avoid searching within, but that is where the solutions really live. We must fine-tune our capacity to go inward, scan our inner wisdom, and *see* solutions. This takes practice. Covering the preferred eye in non–life-threatening situations is a way to access inner focus.

Meier Schneider's story, in his book *Self-Healing: My Life and Vision*, is one of many miracles of recovery. Meier Schneider was born blind, with the congenital condition of cataracts. He was trained to read braille. He grew up in Israel, where a teacher taught him how to gently cover his eyes with his palms and access his inner self. He focused on the warmth of the palms and visualized the healing energy traveling through to the eyes. After months of using this form of stillness and focus, changes began to occur in his ability to see. Objects became more distinct. Schneider now has a California driver's license and a great capacity to look and see. The power to heal existed within his mind.

People commonly are convinced that blindness is irreversible, but for many years surgeons and psychologists have documented cases of congenital blindness in which sight was returned through operations. The most famous of these was reported by von Senden in *Space and Sight: The Perception of Space and Shape in the Congenitally Blind Before and After Operation*, translated by Peter Heath.

One might suppose that these breakthroughs would lead to ecstatic joy for these patients. However, Arthur Zajonc in his book *Catching the Light* reminds us that these formerly blind individuals had developed an accustomed way of navigating as blind people. After an operation of this kind, they suddenly have to include their eyes in negotiating their world, a task that requires new learning and active participation. Learning to see usually evokes a psychological crisis because of a sudden surfacing of the core issues, including hereditary and karmic influences and unresolved life experiences, that underlie the blindness. These issues are activated in the conscious mind and in the unconscious, and if the newly seeing person does not have a support network in place, the process of facing (or not facing) these core issues can be completely overwhelming. Tragically, many of these patients reject their newfound sight. Some have given up altogether and resorted to suicide.

Integrated Vision Therapy offers you a gradual means by which to ignite your imagination and "participate in sight," as Zajonc calls it. Greek literature contains references to the inner light of the body: as early as Plato, sight has been used as a metaphor for "all knowing," says Zajonc, and "eye's fire" is said to be grasping out to make sense of the world. Until science came along and explained vision in terms of the robotic optics of the eye, vision used to be understood philosophically, as a "soul-spiritual" process. Today it has been relegated to the camera analogy of light falling onto the sensitive film called the retina. But "the sober truth remains that vision requires far more than a functioning physical organ," concludes Zajonc. "Without an inner light, without a formative visual imagination, we are blind."

Chapter 8

Renewing
Your Vision

True Self-Expression

Healing wakes up our senses. Our perceptions of ourselves begin to shift. We don't necessarily get rid of the old versions of our earliest videotapes; rather, the new perceptions become more dominant in our view. Imagine a large TV screen with a smaller screen set into one corner. The little screen is the past, which can no longer dominate the whole screen of our enlarged perceptions.

After doing the exercise suggested in chapter 7 of listing the incompletions and distractions in your life and recording your experiences in your journal, patching one eye, and covering both eyes with your palms to relax, you'll find that a new awareness abounds in you. Review your personal journal and summarize any themes you notice. Through your renewed vision, see your former denials, your incompletions, and the aspects of your life that you wish to expand. This new awareness releases many feelings and emotions; you may feel anger, resentment, pain, and guilt. Emerging from perceptual denials opens up your "Pandora's box." Now you are really *seeing* what's present, and facing your truth. At times like this, the transformation process kicks in.

Joe had always wanted to be footloose and fancy-free. Instead, he listened to his father and attended university while his friends went off traveling. The secret desire to go backpacking around the world had always remained with him. He could detect its subconscious presence through the filters of his angry attitude: "If it weren't for my father, I could have traveled a long time ago. If only I hadn't placed my career first, if only I'd stayed single, my dream would have come true." These thoughts were programmed into his psychological videotape library. Although Joe earnestly wanted to change

Joe

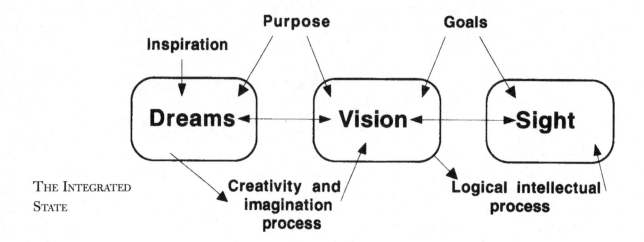

THE INTEGRATED
STATE

his life and follow his passions, most of this debate was happening at the subconscious level, and he began to make choices in his life that would create the opportunity to backpack around the world.

Joe became angry toward his marriage and sabotaged his career. He was in his forties when he lost his job and was served divorce papers on the same day. He was deeply in debt and in a weakened emotional state. As Joe began to use Integrated Vision Therapy daily, his perceptions through his two eyes developed greater degrees of unity and he released much of his genetic rebelliousness and denial patterns. He systematically converted the energy of anger into *seeing* his life through clear filters of passion. Joe reclaimed his love of cooking and fitness. Within six years he was remarried, and he backpacked around the world with his wife.

For many of us, true self-expression was not encouraged when we were growing up. Self-expression and its blocks can stem from the genetic self via the family tree, as well as our experiences of conception, in utero influences, the circumstances of birth, or our perceptions as young children. Our creative capacity to bring out our power through our senses is definitely affected by our parents' child-rearing practices. As children, we were constantly wishing to express our true selves: learning about life through falling down and gently getting up again, touching something hot and getting burned, failing a test and facing rejection, winning an award and feeling proud. These learning experiences can be inhibited or discouraged by overprotective parents, the end result being the stifling of the child's emanating soul expression.

Seeking our power to heal takes us on quite a journey of discovery as adults. Being fully alive and having all our senses firing at peak levels brings forth our internal power. The journey demands that we acknowledge the places where we refuse to be "awake" in our lives. The window to our true passion begins to open, and we begin focusing on completions and on going inward to focus on our real self. This state of being can be called the integrated, or inspired, self. In the flash of a moment, we can convert doing and being into a state of integration and balance. Looking at our loved ones, our children, or spouses, we feel connected. We see them exactly as they are; we are free of bias and judgment, analysis, and the burden of our "critical" self.

I offer my patients an exercise to achieve this form of focus: Imagine you have been given a free holiday to Hawaii. You will be spending three quiet days relaxing in the warm sun and blue-green water. The limousine takes you to a villa with palm trees. Donning your swimsuits, you and your loved one go for a walk through the powdery white sand, into the inviting sea. You put on a mask and snorkel and float in the warm water, looking down into the myriad colors and shapes. Multicolored fish swim around you and the underwater vegetation intrigues you. Your eyes move effortlessly and you see through an open heart. The power behind your eyes surges in inspiration. Your body is relaxed and your imagination is fueled. You are powerful, clear, relaxed, and transformed.

This is the purposeful state of *being* in your vision. You can access it any time—in the subway, in the supermarket, pumping gas into your car, working, driving, or relaxing at home. Achieving this state of being depends on how you filter information from your mind through your eyes.

The creativity within us is a seat of power. The way we express ourselves through movement, writing, drawing, painting, and music all dictate the degree to which we will be able to attain and reside in an inspired, transformed state of self. When these creative components of our beings are suppressed, it deeply affects our self-esteem—the fuel of our power and our spirit. Too often, these creative activities are offered in a competitive context, such as sports and school performance, rather than as an inspirational journey of self-discovery.

Finding self-expression depends on how much we censor our vision with our minds. Our mental protection, that of seeing life in a restricted way, serves to keep our emotional heart-connection intact and safe. As a survival technique we filter what we are seeing through the lens of our own fears, inadequacies, or desires (e.g., my fear of letting my daughter going on the fast ride alone).

In psychological terms, this censoring is called "projection." In photography, we can add a filter to the camera lens to enhance the color of a sunset. It could be midafternoon and yet, with an orange filter in place, the effect would be dusk. Similarly, our personality can create a perceptual filtering mechanism that sees only the negative in a given situation. This enables us to continue to point the finger at the external cause of our problems—something or someone outside ourselves remains unaccountable—and we thus maintain our lofty position of self-righteousness. As long as we practice this form of restricted vision, we shut off our inspired state and hold back our creative self-expression.

John and Maggie

John and Maggie had been married for three years and had a two-year-old son named Matthew. John's visual style of farsightedness and his genetic emotional pattern as determined by iris interpretation didn't at all match Maggie's nearsighted astigmatic looking and her genetic intellectual pattern. This imbalance created the perfect attraction to bring them together, to enable them to move toward balance in their lives.

John's specific filtering habits began with his mother, who was a controlling, intellect-driven person. She complained constantly and spoke in an emotional, overprotective way. Maggie's perceptual challenge began with her father, who had sexually exploited her as a young girl.

Because of withheld resentment and anger toward her father, Maggie looked at men in a distorted, warped (i.e., astigmatic) way. As long as she filtered her perceptions through this protection process, she would not be hurt emotionally by men. She felt safe and untouchable. John, on the other hand, had to block his emotional needs by "spacing out," pushing images away, and developing an unfocused way of being. It seemed as though when he was listening to Maggie talk, his eyes were really focused a hundred miles past her to his first female role model, his mother. His unique filtering strategy eventually resulted in his developing double vision.

The loving attraction John and Maggie had for each other became the stage for healing the respective aspects of their past perceptual filtering. Through Integrated Vision Therapy, John learned to become aware of his projection (his projected critical judgments of his wife), and Maggie systematically removed her filters of defensiveness and the perception that John wanted to attack her. By entering their integrated and inspired selves, John and Maggie were able to enjoy the present rather than resorting to the old projections.

Maggie reclaimed her power by wearing a carefully designed lens prescription that exaggerated her astigmatic blurring. Each time she put on her new eyeglasses, the Integrated Vision Therapy would kick in like a homeopathic remedy. Light pouring through her eye in a specially directed way activated a new, specific focus and an inspirational point of view. Next, by acknowledging her withheld anger, she converted the energy of this anger into focusing on the nurturing role of mothering their first baby, and she found a new passion, playing the piano.

Through special integrated vision practices, John learned how to be focused and present in the moment. His challenge was to learn to stay present with what he was seeing and feeling. At first, this process was challenging; he grew impatient, irritable, and even a little nauseated. In time, however, he could sit six inches from Maggie and truly be with her, *seeing* her the way he had the first time they met.

As adults, we seek classes and seminars to help us unfold the mystery of the imagination. Frederick Frank, in his book *The Zen of Seeing*, uses the practice of drawing to instill the distinction between looking and seeing. In the "flow" state of drawing we can become what we are looking at. I have been applying that same approach to my photography. I am "seeing deeply," as *National Geographic* photographer Dewitt Jones calls it, and merging with what I am seeing. This stirs my sense of connection to life.

Steven

Steven's father was a domineering man who flattened Steven's spirit every time he opened his mouth. As a commercial banker, Steven's father used a visual filter of prestige, image, and clear business logic; he also wished Steven to follow in his footsteps. Steven worked at the bank with his father, but his iris picture revealed that he carried an emotional sensitivity from his mother's genetic package. However, he shut down his emotions at a very early age and was introverted, guarded, and negative. This pulling inward was manifested externally as distress in the form of near-sightedness.

As my patient, Steven was able to become reacquainted with his emotional self and be inspired by it. When he integrated his sensitive side with the gift of his father's logic, Steven was able to focus on leaving his banking career to begin a new profession.

Once that decision had been made, one could hardly recognize Steven. His eyes glowed with the excitement of a two-year-old child. A mischievous energy emanated from his voice as he announced he was becoming a pilot. This was quite a jump for him, but in the integrated state Steven had the inspiration and the power behind his eyes to lift off the runway to a new life.

Drastic Intervention

In the early 1980s, when I developed my twenty-one-day program for renewing vision, my approach was considered quite drastic:

Guidelines for the Twenty-One-Day Program

Obtain a weaker 20/40 prescription.

Wear your lenses only during life-threatening situations.

Eliminate all red meat and dairy products from your diet.

Use no added sugar or foods with sugar.

Use no white-flour products.

Consume no alcohol or bottled or canned prepared drinks.

Use no cigarettes, tobacco, recreational drugs, caffeine drinks, or unnecessary medications.

Wear a patch each day for twenty-one days for a maximum of four hours per day.

Watch no late-night television.

Do not read for pleasure (novels, magazines) or do crossword puzzles.

Take up singing, drawing, painting, sculpting, or writing.

Play vision games each day.

Eat grains, vegetables, legumes, and other healthy foods enriched with sea vegetables such as kelp, kombu, wakame, arame, and hijiki.

Keep a daily diary.

Exercise or move your body for at least fifteen minutes each day.

Today's health-oriented consumers could more easily implement this plan, however, for many people it will take some time to adopt these steps into a new habit pattern.

In my clinical observations, the people who simply adopted this lifestyle, literally overnight, were those who had ongoing daily support. When seeking out a vision therapy optometrist, make sure you also have this support. You may wish to talk with a counselor, minister, or friend about the changes that might occur during the process.

Such drastic intervention as the twenty-one-day program may not always be necessary. Sometimes all we need is a drastic change in attitude. Be careful not to fall into the trap of thinking that the process of integrating your vision requires more *doing*. So often in our lives, we believe we need lots of external busy-ness to bring about changes inside. Many a person I know has thought: "I will diet for a month, exercise vigorously, take night courses, and give up coffee in order to become a whole, healthy person." Integrated vision is a natural unfolding, and each stage of the journey is a natural discovery. You will find that even one perceptual shift can be loaded with new learning and insights that can make you aware.

John needed glasses. As a physician he needed to focus clearly while per- **John**
forming surgery and reading documents. His ophthalmologist had written
a prescription of +2.75. The plus sign indicates farsightedness. This concerned him greatly because of his love for flying airplanes. He needed crisp,
clear *looking* in order to fly, as well as sharp, precise eyesight for surgery.

Normally, the ophthalmological or optometric answer would be quite
simple: a variable-focus lens, or bifocal, which would permit John to focus
sharply at different distances. This approach seems to make perfect sense.
However, I delved deeper into John as a person and spent an extra fifteen
minutes asking him specific questions such as these:

When did you first notice blurry vision?

On a scale of one to ten, how happy are you in your life right now?

What is your daily eating program?

What are your hobbies?

How do you feel about wearing eyeglasses?

These questions elicited a plethora of information. Fifty-four years old,
John had recently begun a physical exercise program, and wondered about
fitness for his eyes and vision. The blurring first occurred during a period
of intense emotional upheaval—the ending of his twelve-year marriage.
Following the divorce he remarried a much younger woman, and they now
had a two-year-old daughter. His new wife was very interested in personal
growth, and had been instrumental in John's opening up to new ideas of
self-development.

On Tuesdays, John was enrolled in counseling classes at the local university to further develop his skill in being with his patients. John had also
begun viewing disease and pathology in a new light. He wanted his patients to take a more active role in their rehabilitation. In John's mind, disease was no longer a death sentence—it was an opportunity to grow.

Armed with this information about John, I was in a strong position to
design an Integrated Vision Therapy program for him. I took the Zen approach. In the West it's known as the K.I.S.S. principle—Keep It Simple,
Sunshine. I suggested that John wear a +1.50 for all his reading activities,
a lens power almost one-half of his first prescription.

I determined his vision fitness to be high enough to manage most of
his close-viewing activities through this lower prescription. In thirty minutes, I taught John how to practice refocusing his attention from his book
to look at far distances, and to keep his eyes moving while he breathed and
blinked. At this stage, his vision fitness for driving or flying without eye-

glasses was about 75 percent, with both his eyes open. John left for vacation with his family to the East Coast. He returned to see me after one month and shared the following story.

While on holiday, he was invited to do rounds in a hospital and to consult on a particular case. At that point, he was asked to perform his own unique surgical procedure. The first thought that ran through his mind was, "I don't have my +2.75 reading glasses. I can't possibly do this surgery." His only choice was to use the awareness gleaned from the Integrated Vision Therapy program: breathe, blink, move the eyes, keep focusing near, far, near, far, and wear the +1.50 "readers."

The surgery was a success. So was his vision fitness. In one month, John had already acquired an additional 20 percent in vision fitness at far distances, which meant he could now fly without eyeglasses. Since that time, he has often performed surgery using the weaker lens prescription.

Julie

Julie wore contact lenses all her waking hours. These contacts permitted excellent eyesight but at the same time entombed the loss of power behind her eyes. As long as she looked through the power of her contact lenses (no matter how much growth occurred in her life), her own innate power was trapped in an addictive process. The contact lens was focusing *for* her, rather than permitting her internal power to blossom.

At age forty, she had been using the contact lenses for eleven years. The power was –3.50 in the right eye and –3.75 in the left. Julie's perception through her left eye was consistently more blurry than her right, in spite of the dioptric difference being only one quarter. This meant that her personal power through Sally was less than through Harry, and potentially the influences from the genetic inheritance of her mother's side of the family was more challenging. Julie informed me that her relationship with her mother had been difficult. (Julie's eye findings compared with how she actually saw through them demonstrates how perceptual adaptations in vision can help explain the background causes of eye difficulty.)

I estimated she could weaken her external lens power by about +1.50. In addition, we decided to weaken the right-eye lens prescription, which would create more blurring in front of her right eye. This would activate more perception through the left eye. This form of lens prescribing is "therapeutic," as opposed to the usual "vision fitness." When Julie put on her new eyeglasses of right eye –0.50 and left –1.25, the therapeutic and homeopathic effect was to stimulate her perception through the left eye and so awaken her feminine power. (Note: This approach is used only when a patient is actively engaged in Integrated Vision Therapy.) In addition to the eyeglasses, she also wore contact lenses of –1.25 for scuba diving and other outdoor activities.

Prior to my meeting Julie, she had been experiencing variable states of depression and anxiety and was taking the antidepressant Prozac. Julie hailed the drug as a miracle worker because of the profound calming effect it had on her. She had never known such periods of blissful peace before.

After beginning Integrated Vision Therapy, Julie received her next wake-up call while traveling overseas, when she was physically attacked and stabbed in the left arm. She ran out of Prozac after she was stabbed, and elected to stop taking it. We discussed the metaphoric link between the left arm and the left eye. Through Integrated Vision Therapy Julie got to the point of attaining the same calmness through her eyes as that she had experienced through the drug. As she put it, "I can now access a natural calm which I could only get before by using Prozac."

Julie now has –0.75 lens power in eyeglasses for each eye and uses them only for driving. Her naked-vision fitness is 78 percent. That is a 50 percent improvement, and her vision is getting better each day. A seven-month period of Integrated Vision Therapy, coupled with many years of personal growth, is bringing about miracle changes in her life and her vision. At forty, her whole life is opening up in front of her. She has more self-confidence and has reclaimed her power behind her eyes. At our last visit she commented, "Being with my naked vision is being with me. I'm not covering myself up."

Seeing Crises Clearly

Take a moment and consider various crises you have dealt with in your life. They may include

Deaths

Emotional or physical abuse

Alcoholism

Separations or divorces

Frequent moves

Pressure at school

Peer or sibling rivalry

Inappropriate career/spouse/lover choices

Lack of money

Illness

Substance abuse

Workaholism

It is usually not easy to *see* clearly during one of these perceived crises. The nature of most Integrated Vision Therapy is to bring these crises to the surface, especially if the unconscious part of your being had to shut down in order to avoid being emotionally hurt—the personality needing to protect the vulnerable soul part of yourself.

As you begin to stimulate an integrated way of being through your eyes and vision, your old avoidances and crises may resurface. From your integrated way of vision and using the biofeedback mechanism of your eyes, you can begin seeing these crises more clearly.

As a nonreader during my primary school years, I experienced plenty of frustration and ridicule. Going to school was, for me, almost a daily crisis. I developed elaborate strategies to compensate for my fear of failure. On days I was to be called before the class to read, make an oral presentation, or recite material, I would feign sickness. I wasn't yet able to face the emotional pain of feeling inadequate and different from my peers. Instead, I focused on what I could be successful in—photography and friendships—and my love for the outdoors. The down side was that in later years more crises continued to surface, this time with the intensities of hurricanes.

I could successfully avoid situations as a child, but as an adult I had to face my crises because they held within them life-threatening consequences. Achieving financial security, raising children, and finding fulfillment were issues I could not avoid, despite my fear of failure. Fortunately, my wake-up calls brought me rich learning experiences, and I weathered the storms. I chose to see crises as opportunities to renew my vision.

National Geographic photographer Dewitt Jones advises: "When you see something pleasing you wish to photograph, consider the object or view from many vantage points. The final photograph may have as many as five to fifteen other right answers. There are many creative solutions to arrive at a final rendering." In life there are many ways of seeing crises clearly. It's a matter of opening your eyes to these possibilities, these different points of view.

True *seeing* is responding to that gift and challenge in every crisis. Going with the flow becomes the opportunity. Most of nature is designed according to this principle. As a fisherman I observe the waxing and waning of the tides. As a photographer I enjoy the sunrises and sunsets. I can't control what time the sun is going to go down for me to get the perfect picture. I need to plan and be prepared, as the Boy Scout motto states.

Dealing with eye conditions and vision challenges requires the same flexibility. At times, the Integrated Vision Therapy approaches I've been suggesting work well. In other situations, a more allopathic solution (one of incorporating surgery or drugs) may be necessary. As a rule, I use allopathic forms of vision care to help me define the specific challenges, and then use Integrated Vision Therapies to respond to them. Sometimes I weave the two together. Each situation is unique.

Mary

Mary had already lessened her dependency on glasses for far-away looking. When she was in her late fifties, her vision began to get dim and blurry again. Her ophthalmologist diagnosed her as having cataracts in both eyes and recommended an operation. Mary decided to go ahead with surgery that would put a lens implant in each eye. She also chose to use certain components of Integrated Vision Therapy prior to and following the surgery.

I assisted Mary in designing a self-healing audiotape, one that dealt with all her fears of blindness and taught her how to activate her own self-healing powers. She used this tape as a tool to increase the healing of the eye tissue surrounding the lens implant. Her response was excellent. In just a few weeks, her eyes could see very well through the lens implants and Mary's visual confidence and optimism returned.

Nadine

As a youngster, Nadine had a lazy right eye. Her father was absent most of her childhood, and her eyes became crossed. Nadine's eyes were a place of great vulnerability.

An emotional individual, she carried much anger and resistance. Through her teenage years she avoided the challenges being presented through her eyes, but her underlying desire to be a whole person kept presenting eye-messages to her. At first the messages were minimal, but so were her intention and commitment. She paid only casual attention to the subtle signals. She was losing more sight in her right eye.

When she was twenty-five, Nadine began applying vision therapy measures, but she had not fully committed to changing her life path. It took a full-blown crisis for her to begin responding to what her eyes had been telling her. The ophthalmologist couldn't diagnose a specific condition, but the failing sight in her right eye was enough to indicate the need for exploratory surgery.

After much deliberation, Nadine decided to follow through. The surgery and subsequent tests revealed no malignancy, and in the following weeks, her eyes continued to heal as she applied colored light and palming.

After a while, though, Nadine became focused again on her career plans. She began to forget to take care of herself, to make time for her needs being reflected metaphorically through her right eye. I had advised her to slow down, nurture herself, make time for her relationship with her boyfriend, and open her heart to what was important for her rather than just focusing on the survival needs of making ends meet. After a recurrent infection in her eye and a short hospital stay, she chose to respond by following the more integrated approach of taking time for her self-healing. She created a daily program of using color, imagining the regeneration of the optic nerve, and expanding her field of vision to bring this new awareness into action.

Imaging Visual Wellness

You can use the following material to design your own audiotape narrative to induce healing by positive reinforcement. Include appropriate commentaries for your unique eye condition in your narrative.

Make yourself comfortable. Lie down, or sit on the floor or in a chair. Begin breathing in an integrated way. Let your eyes close and become relaxed throughout your body as the audiotape begins. Here is a suggested narrative:

With each breath I take, I feel more and more relaxed. I feel my whole body letting go of muscle tension and tightness. As I breathe I feel my active mind becoming still. I sense peace throughout my body. As I breathe I bring the calmness of a sunset into my awareness. I hear seagulls overhead and the lapping of the ocean waves. With each breath I take I see the vivid colors of the setting sun. The oranges, reds, and pinks look vibrantly alive. As I breathe I feel more and more relaxed. I use this tranquil sensation to let go of my daily challenges and to bring my vision back into balance. With each breath I take, I become more and more and more relaxed. I feel the tightness of my body muscles melting like snow on a sunny day. I breathe, breathe, breathe, and let go. It feels so good to just let go. My life is becoming simpler as I let this relaxation move through every muscle spindle in my body. I feel the tightness of my controlling personality fading into the distance, like an eagle soaring into the sky. As I breathe I bring this relaxed feeling to my eyes. I feel the muscles around my eyes beginning to unwind, like a tight spring that is being released. It feels wonderful to let my eyes assume their normal relaxed posture. I feel a warm sensation moving through my eyes, like the summer sun's rays beaming down through them. With each relaxed breath I take, I feel the vitality and aliveness returning to my eyes. I feel my eyes are beautiful and clear. . . ."

Now your audiotape should include one or more of the following specific images to help you with your unique eye problem. Create your statement in the first person, beginning with "I."

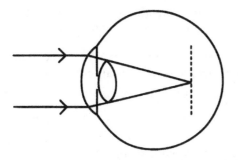

For near-sightedness

Imagine looking into your eyeball where the musculature is relaxing, your eyeball is shortening, and the cornea is flattening. Visualize your eyes focusing outward into space.

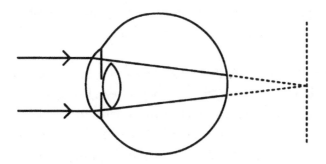

For far-sightedness

Imagine that your eyeball is elongating and your focusing muscle is able to change shape with greater speed and facility. Imagine focusing more easily at closer distances.

Imagine a more spherical cornea. Breathe into the cornea and the lens, thus reducing the tension of the muscles surrounding your eyes.

For astigmatism

Visualize these muscles changing their tension to allow the return of accurate alignment. Imagine looking through your eyes and viewing the world two-eyed, looking straight ahead, and with both eyes working together.

For a lazy eye

Imagine yellow and orange light coming into your so-called lazy eye. Let go of the limiting perception that this eye is weak. Have the light stimulate the back of the eye in the area of the retina known as the fovea. Imagine

For crossed- or walleyes

135

yourself being nestled in the groove at the back of the eye known as the macula. Feel the macula and fovea being stimulated and awakened.

To awaken two-eyed perception

If you had difficulty seeing two thumbs when you looked past your out-stretched thumb, imagine you can successfully see two thumbs in your mind. Continue your integrated breathing, and visualize that the retina of each eye is willing to receive incoming light. Through your breath, awaken your foveal sensitivity by sending your heartfelt loving energy to the foveas and retinas of each eye to heighten your ability for two-eyed vision. Picture the feminine and masculine aspects of your nature that you wish to manifest in your life.

For corneal dystrophy

Consider the vital nutrients flowing to the cornea, and this magnificent biosphere-shaped structure regenerating. Picture the cornea becoming clearer and clearer, like a freshly cleaned window.

For keratoconus

Create the image of a half-sphere. Pretend you can massage your cornea back into this perfect spherical shape without any discomfort or pain. Feel your power surging back into your heart and eyes.

For glaucoma

Feel the ease with which the watery fluids in your eyes can drain from the front (behind the cornea) to the back of your eye. Let all the pressures of your life drain away as you breathe and remain perfectly relaxed. See your optic nerve regenerating through the nutrients in the healthy food you are putting into your body. Imagine your eye pressures lowering each day as you relax and let integrated vision return to your life. Pretend you are back in your eye doctor's office and notice the surprised look on his or her face as you are told that your eye pressures have dropped. Smile at your success.

For cataracts

Focus your attention on the lens of your eye, the structure behind the pupil. Imagine the last time you cleaned a window. A cataract is like an un-washed, cloudy window. With each breath you take, imagine that the window to your vision is becoming cleaner and more transparent. Imagine that the debris in the lens of your eye represents the unfinished clutter of your life. As you complete the unfinished busy-ness of your existence, you can restore the clarity of your lenses.

For eye floaters

Consider the vitreous jelly of your eyes behind the lens and in front of the retina. After examining projects and situations that are still unnecessarily floating around in your life, picture your eye floaters dissolving like butter in a frying pan. If you have a serious physical condition such as diabetes, in which floaters are common, permit a feeling of wellness to permeate your entire body during this practice. Feel the energizing vitamins, minerals, and antioxidants from your healthy diet encouraging your total well-being.

Imagine that the detachment is like a flap that has turned upward. While continuing your feeling of relaxation, envision taking the flap and reinserting it into the retina or vitreous. Ponder where you may have detached yourself from some vital aspect of your life, or from your dreams and visions. Where has your survival-based personality taken you away from your soul? **For retinal or vitreous detachments**

Enjoy your relaxed state and reflect on this feeling of total well-being. Say: "It is safe for me to feel, feel, feel, feel, feel, and feel." Imagine your healthy blood is carrying rich sources of nutrients to your retina. Feel your damaged tissue regenerating in each moment of relaxation. In this state of being, you have the potential to activate the extraordinary healing powers of your brain and mind. Feel your retinal tissue coming alive. Let the inactive rods and cones begin to function with renewed spirit and enthusiasm. **For other retinal conditions**

Feel yourself flowing through life with ease. Begin this journey in your brain, where the optic nerve begins its downward, winding journey, through the visual radiations, to the back of the eye. See this path as a long ski slope. As the blood and nerves energetically flow, feel your optic nerves becoming stimulated, as if they were waking from a deep sleep. Where in your life have you sacrificed moving forward? Where do you feel stuck? Commit to resolving these situations to reclaim your natural, healthy vision. **For optic nerve conditions**

Travel to the back of your eye, to the central depression in the retina. Breathe, recognizing that you are supercharging your maculae with delicious whole grains, such as brown rice and millet. These grains feed the necessary B-complex vitamins to the macula. What part of your existence has begun to deteriorate? Is your vision of this situation real, or is it an illusionary perception based on fear? As you develop your capacity to relax deeply, let your mind discover new solutions to these challenges. **For macular degeneration**

Get in touch with your hidden anger and frustration. Make a wide yawn and feel the tension in your body, face, and eye muscles floating away like a puffy cloud in the sky. Meditate on those aspects of your life where you have not forgiven others. Begin to bring deep-heart focus to these situations. Resolve to complete the cycles of these past events that have resulted **For any eye condition ending in "-itis"**

137

in your choosing to hold onto your past anger. If the anger you feel is meant to punish others, ask yourself if it is really hurting *them* for *you* to hold onto your anger, or is it only blocking you from getting on with the enjoyment of your life?

Now continue with the narrative:

I am clear that within my loving, compassionate heart is the ability for me to heal my eyes and my vision. I can feel my clear purpose being manifested on the earth plane. My vision of my life is becoming clearer each day as I remain relaxed and allow my eyes to see clearly. As I breathe, I feel a warmth moving from my heart to my eyes. I sense a deeper level of integration of my Harry and Sally perceptions.

As you end the meditation, slowly become aware of your body. Blink your eyelids, open your eyes, and return to being in the room. Let the light in, feeling refreshed in your eyes. After taking a few minutes to adjust to your relaxed state, continue with your day. Your adventurous journey toward clear vision continues.

Chapter 9

Life's Opportunities

Reclaiming Your Power— Your Naked Vision

Contact lenses are the vision marvel of the twentieth century. From their beginning incarnation, when users had to build up wearing time, to the convenience of throwaways, contact lenses have taken their toll on human consciousness. The less we pay attention to the miracle of our naked vision, the more visually unconscious we become. The razor-edge sharpness created through contact lenses creates a forced focus. The contact lenses act as an external power that deprives us of the opportunity to generate our own vision. We assume a protected place behind the barrier of lenses, between our hearts and what we see in the world.

Contact lenses are the most sophisticated form of visual unconsciousness. Having stated this, let me add that I am not against contact lenses. On the contrary, I view all lenses in a similar way: They must be prescribed in a manner that considers the whole person.

Think about it for a moment: In most cases when we suspect there is something wrong with our eyes, we give our power over to the eye doctor, who literally decides how we are to see in the future. The doctor's biases and prejudices are impregnated into the lens prescription, thus removing our choices. Most of the time lens prescriptions for both contacts and eyeglasses are too strongly focused. Perhaps in looking clearly through these lens prescriptions we *see* less because we have to participate less. Our eyes don't need to focus, so we in turn don't need to face ourselves intimately. This is especially true for contact lenses. We pop them in in the morning, and for the rest of the day we busily go on with our life, not giving a second thought to our vision. At least with eyeglasses we can take them off, rest our eyes, and face the fears and denials presented through our naked vision.

The vision-care industry has perpetuated the belief that we need to have 20/20 vision in order to be able to drive and not get into accidents. This is a safe approach. Most states and provinces, however, give a 16 percent vision leeway for driving. This means that we can drive with an 84 percent level of usable vision. A loss of clearness of 16 percent does not dramatically impact reaction times in driving.

Many eye doctors assert that we need 20/20 vision in order to see a child crossing the street, but in fact the peripheral vision of the retina is much more sensitive than the fovea in catching movement at the edges of our field of vision—especially in the presence of 16 percent blurring. Why? Because the slight blurring of eyesight forces us to be more present and aware of what is happening. Remember, the focusing of light on the retina permits more feeling. This awareness of what is around us broadens our perspective.

The disempowering effect of a lens prescription that is too strong is to create separation. Have you ever put on your new eyeglasses and felt as if the whole world were farther away? Or the surface you are walking on seems to jump at you, or curve like a flying carpet? This initial perception is your brain adjusting to your way of *looking* through your new lens prescription. Through that illusionary veil, the world appears to be clear. Yet the heart knows differently—the world still *feels* unsafe. Our perceptions are still fearful and we continue to disengage our inherent power. Our jobs, relationships, business ventures, and parenting responsibilities are all seen through our artificial lenses of prejudice and protection.

The solution is to gradually rekindle your own power. Gradually, your lens prescriptions can be weakened, allowing you time to see through progressively less outside influence. You begin to make your own choices. As you reaccess the power behind your eyes, life seems to slow down. You take time to smell the flowers and find yourself really listening to what people say. The internal self-talk is replaced with the feeling of stillness, much like an early morning sunrise. A peaceful feeling radiates throughout your body.

For those of us who have worn lens prescriptions for many years, exploring our naked vision offers a state of enlightenment and being intimately focused on the self. This inward focus exposes vulnerability and fears. Spend time at home enjoying and *being* in your naked vision. Many of us have forgotten how to experience what simply is—to feel vulnerable, to do less, to begin seeing through your other body senses and feelings. Let the muscles around the eyes relax, then let your hands explore a familiar object. Experience what it is rather than what you think it is.

The more we give our power away to someone or something outside of ourselves—the boss, the job, the firm, your wife, husband, mother, father—the higher the probability that these distorted perceptions become physically apparent in the refractive measurements of the eyes.

Since the 1950s, vision therapy optometrists have used a special instrument called a retinoscope to observe and measure these mind/power influences upon eye function. While you are contemplating a particular thought, the vision therapy optometrist examines the reflection of the retina as seen in the pupil of your eye. A single thought, feeling, or emotion can modify the intensity and degree of this reflection. A fear response can alter the perceived reflex by a significant amount.

If you arrive at your eye doctor's office full of fear, your new lens prescription will probably reflect the emotional state you were in at that time. Ask your optometrist to perform your vision examination without eye drops, which paralyze your eye's focusing mechanism. (Paralysis of your power to focus clearly during the examination results in you having to wear a stronger addictive lens prescription and feeling less powerful.)

How much of your power did you surrender to the eye doctor during the vision examination? Were you fully relaxed? Before your next eye examination begins, take a few moments to breathe and shift your focus in different directions. Also do this during the testing procedures. Ask for the minimum lens prescription for 20/20, or better still, use a 20/20 lens prescription only for driving and during other life-threatening activities. If you spend most of your day reading close up, ask for a pair of eyeglasses that are 20/40, which is 84 percent vision fitness (or 16 percent blur), or 20/50, which is 76 percent vision fitness (or 20–25 percent blur).

You visit an eye doctor because you want to help your vision and regain visual clarity. Vision-therapy–oriented optometrists or behavioral optometrists can sometimes assist you with a more holistic approach. These doctors will take the measurements of your eyes so that you can reclaim or restimulate the power behind your eyes. The most important step is to break the habit and control of that part of the personality, the ego-survival state, that locks you into believing you need strong lenses to attain a perfect 20/20 and saps your internal capacity to be in control.

Sam

Sam, in his early twenties, had been told by his ophthalmologist that his eyesight was not good enough for him to be eligible for the police academy. He was devastated. His grades were good and his body physically fit, but his eyes were not clear. He began researching the corneal laser procedure for "correcting" nearsightedness, and intuitively knew that it was not for him. By chance he visited an optometrist with whom I had been collaborating, and heard about the vision-fitness approach I was using.

As in 80 to 90 percent of all cases, Sam's prescription included an astigmatic component. I read the hidden message printed out in his lens prescription. Sam's personality-driven state, as represented by his right-eye perception (Harry), was too dominant over his Sally connection to his heart. Sam was placing himself under too much external strain by studying and continually aligning his eyes. His life lacked balance. His excessive work regimen and the demands of becoming a policeman were driving Sam's focus too far inward, at the expense of his creative life.

In spite of the external demands for clarity, Sam reconnected to his internal power, kept himself in focus, used the eye-mind relaxation procedures of covering his eyes, used full spectrum lighting, focused far away, and shifted his visual attention around the room. These exercises eventually resulted in improved eyesight. Within three months, Sam passed the police academy's visual examination and is now studying to be a policeman.

Nearsightedness— Reach Out Fearlessly to the Future

Nearsightedness, also known as shortsightedness or myopia, affects sixty to eighty million Americans alone, according to a 1994 study by Zadnik and associates. Defined conventionally, nearsightedness results from an eyeball that is too long, thus forcing light to focus in front of the retina. From an Integrated Vision Therapy perspective, nearsightedness is a pulling in of one's perceptual reality. Early symptoms include slight, blurry faraway vision, such as seeing blurry letters on the board at school, blurry freeway signs, or blurry images on a movie screen. Measuring the eyeball itself may not reveal nearsightedness, because pulling in of space begins with the thought "I don't know how to handle what's out there—my world is too confusing. I feel too much when I look beyond myself. I can't cope with what's out there. I feel safe when I focus mentally inward. I will feel less by thinking more. Give me a book to read. I'll master this computer program. I'll take courses at university. I'll excel at school."

Nearsightedness is a practiced form of looking; it disengages our feelings and our connection to what is happening outside. The more we project inward, the more unresolved fear builds up inside us. Through nearsighted vision and compensatory prescription lenses, we create a zone of comfort and define this as our life.

Breaking this cycle means facing our fears and reaching out. You may be able to use a lens prescription weaker than 20/40 for close-up work such as reading, working at a computer, or sewing. Check with your optometrist.

Read for short periods without eyeglasses. Spend safe time in your naked vision. Look at your environment, clean your house, or go for a walk. Move around your home experiencing your blur and remembering that the blur varies according to the distance between your eyes and the object you are looking at. The Far Eye-C chart is an excellent way to monitor your level of blur and clarity and to watch how the level fluctuates. This variable blur is a measure of your ability to let go of your habitual pattern of looking. Without a lens prescription, you can train yourself to be farsighted: relax, move outside your comfort zone, deal with your fears and frustrations as they surface. Whenever you feel pressure in or around your eyes or when your eyes are tired, palm your eyes. Write about your experience in your journal.

As you experiment with life in your naked vision, you will probably be amazed at how much you can actually see, especially in familiar environments such as your home. You recognize shapes, color, size, distance, and texture. As long as you don't have to focus on details, you can enjoy the freedom and power of your naked vision. Begin looking into your future, reacquainting yourself with vision that feels focused through your heart.

Nearsighted people often have similar characteristics. The individual caricature of the intellectual, introverted, and precise person springs to mind. Careers such as engineering, accounting, or computer science seem to suit the nearsighted personality. But what happens to nearsighted people's perception of work and life once their perceptions change and their vision improves? Quite often they wish to change such aspects of their life as careers or relationships. This is a reminder that the power behind your eyes is more than what is measured by your lens prescription. Your total being is the power behind your eyes.

Farsightedness—
Focus Passionately on the Now

Farsightedness is also called hyperopia or longsight. Typically, the farsighted person can see far away but finds that reading small type is a great challenge. In many cases, between the ages of forty and sixty-five, farsighted persons also begin noticing a blurring of faraway details such as those on road signs. At this point, the eye doctor might recommend bifocals or separate glasses for faraway and close-up looking.

From a Western medical perspective, farsightedness means that the eyeball is too short—the person is less able to focus the incoming light onto the retina. Like nearsightedness, farsightedness is not a fixed or permanent phenomenon. From a behavioral perspective, farsightedness varies according to

143

our attention to detail (mind focus) as well as with emotional and nutritional factors. It appears that eating sugary foods, for example, can profoundly affect a farsighted person's ability to focus. The integrated way of dealing with farsightedness is to examine aspects of the person's intimate life such as relationships, family, and career. Farsightedness is a gift that can enable a person to deal with unresolved anger and issues of intimacy.

In evaluating farsightedness, I look at where individuals can function well and where they are challenged. Devoting close-up focus on aspects of their lives that are near and dear to them presents the opportunity to grow. If you are farsighted, begin to identify any unresolved close-up aspects of your life while using weaker lens prescriptions or spending time in your naked vision. Write down your frustrations about specific situations.

If you use a lens prescription for distance viewing, as when watching TV or driving, start training your naked vision to sharpen its focus and use the Far Eye-C chart as a way to verify your improvements. If you use reading glasses, you will find that they are becoming too strong. Ask for a weaker prescription. These recommendations also apply to the "short-arm" syndrome, or middle-aged difficulties with reading.

Remember, your skill is reaching out to life with great gusto and passion. As you develop flexible focusing on the intimate aspects of your life, your own power will reemerge. Choices that you made earlier in life may seem less important or necessary now. Rediscover the kindness you feel through your heart for all living things on Earth. This is the true power of seeing.

Astigmatism

In most cases, astigmatism will accompany either far- or nearsightedness. In nearsightedness, keep the astigmatism correction for the first weaker lens prescription. For farsightedness, the astigmatism correction can be partially reduced on the first lens prescription change.

For the three illustrations of various types of astigmatism, use the eye crossing and uncrossing modes of looking and seeing outlined in chapter 3. Bring A on top of B to create an image like C. Start by practicing whichever illustration is easiest for you, then progress to the more difficult ones. Make sure that the letters and lines are as clear as possible.

Crossed or Wandering Eyes

Strabismus is the name given to eye conditions that involve an eye turning in. You may hear your doctor calling the condition *esotropia* for crossed eyes or *exotropia* for wandering eyes. Beware of falling prey to the assump-

Vertical Astigmatism
(More blurry in vertical)

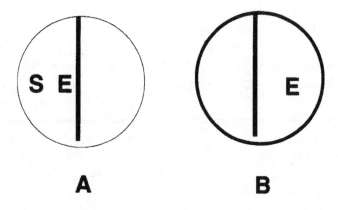

A   B

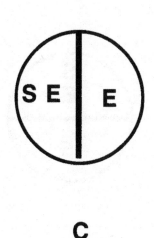

C

Horizontal Astigmatism
(More blurry in horizontal)

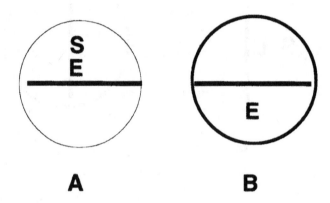

A   B

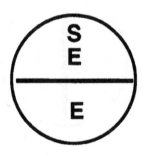

C

Oblique Astigmatism
(More blurry in obliques)

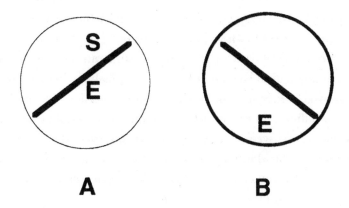

A   B

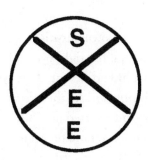

C

tion that these eye conditions are always due to a faulty muscle in the eye. Through the vehicle of your eyes, your mind is attempting to communicate a message to you about your vision. The crossed eye is a turning inward of that eye's perception; a walleye is a wandering off of that eye's perception. Both conditions make it difficult for your vision to stay integrated in a two-eyed perceiving way.

Matthew

Little Matthew, aged three, visited me because of a noticeable inward turning of his right, or Harry, eye. You might guess which parent brought him in to see me—yes, his mother. The metaphoric "eye printout" of his father's side of the family showed a tendency to shut out that relationship. His perceptual adaptation was one of turning his feelings inward about something he was seeing in relationship to men. I asked his mother about Matthew's father, and she nonchalantly informed me that he had walked out on them three weeks earlier. This corresponded almost exactly to the first occurrence of Matthew's crossed eye. You might think that the eye condition and the father's absence is too much of a coincidence; however, I have seen case upon case like this one.

A word of caution: Not all strabismus is so closely related to life events. The predisposition for the eye condition probably exists long before the eye is seen to deviate; the life experience sets off a trigger for the "turning in" or "wandering out" to happen. This can take the form of an illness, accident, emotional upset, or too many demands for achievement. Each case is unique and full of its own surprises.

In the case of Matthew, if the right eye had wandered out, the interpretation would have been a little different. This type of eye says: "I am going to just let go and push outward in this situation." The inward-eye child would probably be more introverted about his deepest feelings, not showing much emotion in such a traumatic event as his father walking out on the family. In the wandering-outward eye condition, the child could be overtly emotional about the situation and behave in an unruly way.

In most cases of crossed or wandering eyes, ophthalmologists advocate a survival approach of correcting faulty muscles. The usual treatment for these conditions is either the surgical shortening or lengthening of one of the six muscles in each eye, or a combination of surgery with an exercise program. Richard Kavner and other behavioral optometrists recognize that surgery produces a high rate of cosmetic success in that the eyes appear straighter, but it may not produce a higher level of two-eyed integration. Alternatively, vision therapy encourages the eyes not only to look more aligned but also to work better together. Optometrists who practice vision therapy will outline a vision exercise program for correcting crossed eyes or walleyes. To improve your vision in the case of inward (crossed) or outward (wall) eyes, you can ask your optometrist to weaken the lens prescription to the exact point where you are challenged to use both eyes together. In the case of a lazy eye, the lens prescription for 20/25 (or as measured in the eye) is maintained to give you the maximum chance of enhancing your perception through that eye. Use sticky tape over the lens of your other eye to act as a translucent patch. Patch for no more than four hours and only in non–life-threatening situations.

The results of this kind of program can be life changing. Improvement in two-eyed vision affects a person's whole personality and thus his or her behavior toward family and loved ones and in the world. Improving two-eyed vision involves much more than just straightening a pair of eyes.

What if You Already Have 20/20?

Perfect 20/20 vision does not guarantee that the two eyes will successfully integrate the Harry and Sally perceptions. I see many patients who have excellent 20/20 eyesight—they don't wear glasses, and on the surface it would appear they have good vision—but they have no depth of multidimensional vision, the vision that links your soul and your personality. These individuals also manifest a particular visual style of relating to the world. They will be slightly farsighted and reveal an outward-reaching aggressive and artistic nature. Some are poor readers who lean toward working with their hands in their professional careers. This does not mean that they are any less intellectually endowed than the nearsighted person who excels at academic activities. The difference is in their way of visually processing information.

Farsighted people with 20/20 vision see more globally, and so find it difficult to focus on small details. If the social and political community at large does not understand this and accept them, these people often demonstrate antisocial behavior. They may adopt addictive ways of living. In the worst-case scenario, they might resort to crime.

Behavioral optometrists Stan Kaseno, Roger Dowis, Joel Zaba, and others have pioneered inspiring research in which they found that the juvenile-delinquent population they studied tended, by and large, to have good eyesight but poorly developed perceptual skills. They had difficulty in making shape and size discrimination and sequencing verbal and written thoughts, and they often confused left and right.

The findings suggest that these young people have somehow developed a restricted perceptual way of seeing. They find it arduous to switch points of view. Their vision lacks flexibility and synthesis. Their learning style makes them unresponsive to the way programs offered by the traditional educational system are taught. They learn better by working from global to specific.

Children who are labeled "learning disabled" have similar difficulties. Visually, they tend to be a little farsighted and to reverse letters and words. These are dyslexic behaviors. Poor attention span is quite common among learning-disabled children, and they don't retain or comprehend very well. These behaviors are all related to incomplete or distorted visual perception.

When the educational approach is modified to parallel these children's visual and learning style, reading becomes much easier for them. If they are forced to learn without first developing visual skills, school becomes arduous and their self-esteem suffers. A significant percentage of juvenile delinquents have a history of learning problems. One could speculate that perhaps this is the youngsters' way of gaining attention. They focus through their personality and display anger, fear, or both.

Stan Kaseno, who pioneered vision therapy for juvenile delinquents with visual challenges, found that their visual-processing style could be broadened. His most satisfying discovery was the dramatically lower re-cidivism rate following the implementation of a vision therapy program. Young offenders who undertook vision therapy were less likely to run into trouble once released from the court system. From this outcome one can infer that these young people became more responsible once their vision is calibrated to their heart and feelings. They focused on life through new eyes. This is just one example of how people with "good eyesight" have benefited from vision therapy.

Your concentration will be higher, you will read more efficiently and maintain higher comprehension, and even your sports performance can be improved if you work to gain a higher level of vision fitness in the presence of 20/20 vision. (With the advent of computer software that can generate random-dot stereograms, public awareness of multidimensional vision is growing.) Practice your eye crossing or uncrossing on the illustration on page 59 until the image begins to emerge from the background. This can be very beneficial in helping build two-eyed stamina. It is a standard vision therapy activity for enhancing the brain's capacity to stay integrated under varying degrees of daily distress.

If you now have 20/20 vision, you no doubt want to maintain this crisp vision throughout your future years. In spite of increasing lifespans, oph-thalmologists and optometrists alike keep telling their patients that middle-

or old-age sight deficiencies are inevitable. This negative programming can be replaced with eye activities for maintaining 20/20 vision. Regular exercising of the eye muscles and controlling them with your brain can do wonders if you work on computers or do a lot of desk work. Exercising your eyes is just like maintaining the other parts of your body: the more you stimulate the muscles, the better your vision fitness and the more you can accomplish. Begin the two-eyed games from chapter 3 as a daily practice. Palm your eyes when they become tired. Above all, believe in wellness and the innate ability your body has to communicate exactly what it needs.

Eye Diseases—What Can I Do?

The onset of an eye-disease condition usually means your eye is responding to a specific command from your soul. Your soul is saying to your dominating personality: "Please include me." When are you going to pay attention to your red warning light? Are you going to wait for it to begin flashing desperately before you notice it? Perhaps you will need an exploding light, as one of my patients recently described it. She had been so obsessed with her university studies and with holding down a legal secretarial job that a major catastrophe had to occur before she *saw*! She was adjusting her new halogen desk lamp and looked into the bulb for a short moment. The intensity of the light caused retinal burns, and she had massive afterflashes and fireworks in her eyes. Only when she took the time to look deeply at her life situation did she see the dis-ease—the precursor to disease—in her life. She gave up her studies and quit her job to take a fresh look at her vision for the future.

For twenty years I have been chronicling the metaphoric link of eye conditions with the way patients lead their lives. Glaucoma is indicative not only of pressure buildup in the eye but of mental pressure in the person's life. Retinal detachments could be a report of the person's detachment from certain aspects of life. The part of the retina where the detachment occurs might give us a clue to the part of life that he or she is wishing to not see or be attached to. Is the detachment necessary because of excessive attachments in the person's life? Macular degeneration is a loss of focus on the central theme of life. It is quite common to see the onset of this condition at about the time a person enters retirement age. The patients I have seen tend to have lost their zest for living. This condition also appears when there has been a loss of a loved one.

Perhaps you have a sight-threatening eye disease or you have just been informed of some terrible-sounding condition of your eyes. Your mind immediately paints the worst picture: "I am going to go blind!" The doctors usually suggest a sight-saving surgical procedure or a medication that can prevent the condition from getting to the point where destructive damage occurs in the eye tissue. It is important to ask yourself: "Why has this condition manifested in my eye in the first place? What can I learn from this experience?" Avoid the trap of thinking that all you have to do is get the condition fixed. Whatever the "problem" is, a useful solution can direct you to higher levels of consciousness if you are ready.

How does one become ready to learn from eye conditions? First, familiarize yourself with the name of the eye disease. The most common eye conditions are listed in table 1. Identify the part of the eye that is affected. In macular degeneration for example, the macula of the eye, which is situated on the part of the retina surrounding the fovea, is affected.

Using table 2, visualize the eye anatomy in order to begin a dialogue with these parts of your eyes. Think about the potential metaphoric connection between the eye condition and the message your mind is attempting to communicate to you. Write down the day and time when you first began to have symptoms. These may have included blurring or double vision, headaches, or loss of vision in particular areas of your seeing. When did the doctor first make a diagnosis? What was going on in your life at that time? This writing exercise will help you understand the various correlations that will emerge from this study. Your eyes are simply attempting to wake you up to a new awareness and assist you in being more visually present. Keep this goal in mind and your journey will become more exciting and worthwhile.

Now that you have identified the lifestyle correlations and you understand the anatomy and the eye condition, you are ready to add your eye doctor's recommendations. In the case where the physician says that nothing more can be done for your eyes, the complementary approach becomes the primary healing. In those cases of eye diseases where medications or surgical intervention is prescribed, adding complementary approaches enhances the possibility of increased wellness.

The complementary approaches allow you to be a more active participant in your own healing program. Otherwise, you may feel entirely at the mercy of your eye doctor. For instance, a patient of mine was recently informed by her ophthalmologist that her glaucoma condition had progressed far enough to affect her visual field, and there was a strong possibility that she would go blind in that eye. We had begun using complementary procedures involving colored-light therapy, visualization, and therapeutic food supplementation, and the visual field loss had not constricted any further since she had become involved in her own healing program. She felt better about herself and her capacity to continue the self-healing, but at her

TABLE 1. YOUR EYE CONDITION "THE GIFT"	TRADITIONAL DIAGNOSIS	WHAT YOUR MIND AND EYES ARE TRYING TO TELL YOU	NEW THINKING	COMPLEMENTARY ACTION
Nearsightedness	Eyeball too long, cornea too steep.	You are afraid to see what's out there. You are pulling too far inward to "self."	Reach out with clear purpose. Begin taking risks.	Modified lens prescriptions. Relaxation with vision games which allow "being" more than "doing."
Farsightedness	Eyeball too short. Lens not powerful enough.	You are pushing space and people away. Break out and be independent.	Focus, be inward and close to people, life, and situations. Learn cooperation.	Modified lens prescription. Vision games to focus and center.
Astigmatism	Cornea (or lens) not equally curved.	There is a distortion of one part of your visual reality.	Begin identifying past warped perceptions.	Focus on vision games to see specific visual orientations.
Vitreous floaters	Debris in vitreous.	There are incompletions floating around in your life.	Melt away the past warped perceptions.	Imagery and color balancing.
Glaucoma	Pressure in your eye.	There is internal pressure.	Modify your lifestyle to increase relaxation and recreation.	Color balancing, nutrition, and visualization.
Eye crossing or turning	Weak eye muscles.	Life is too much for you to integrate.	Heal relationships with parents and see straight to the point.	Vision Fitness Training, light therapy.
Macular degeneration	You're getting old.	You no longer see the point to living.	Reclaim your purpose. See exciting new possibilities.	Color balancing, visualization, light therapy.
Retinal detachment	Retina has lifted.	You feel separate. You are losing touch with outside/inside reality.	Feel part of life's family. Commit to specific future plans— SEE rather than LOOK.	Imagery, nutritional approach. Nutrition, imagery, color light therapy.
Cataract	Cloudy lens.	You are clouding and blocking out—avoiding.	Become aware of the influences that block your personal vision.	Color balancing, visualization, psycho-emotional release.
Corneal conditions	Weakness.	You see pain. You are blocking off personal power.	Feel powerful from within— connect to life's power.	Color light therapy, movement exercise.
Optic atrophy	"Dead" nerve.	You are self-destructing. Part of you and your life is dying.	Stimulate your aliveness. Revitalize your life's vision.	Release anger with specific relaxation techniques.
Iritis	Inflammation of the iris.	You have anger toward family members.	Allow resentment to flow away from you. Feel your heart open. Let love flow to all you see.	Visualization.

TABLE 2. EYE PARTS	LOCATION AND FUNCTION	HEALING METAPHOR	VITAMINS, MINERALS, AND HERBS	FOODS
Cornea	Front surface. Changes light; tears flow across it.	Power and/or struggle.	Vitamin A and healthy tears.	Dark green and yellow fruits and vegetables, egg yolks.
Pupil	Black part of the eye. Responds to light.	Window of stimulation/relaxation—dealing with light.	Full-spectrum light.	Sunlight, full-spectrum fluorescent or incandescent color-corrected light.
Iris	Colored part of the eye. Its muscle action facilitates pupil-changing size.	Transgenerational map of family influences—inner mind.	Full-spectrum light.	Sunlight, full-spectrum fluorescent or incandescent color-corrected light.
Lens	Snuggled behind pupil Increase in shape permits a sharper focus of light.	Focus and intention—flexibility and capacity to metabolize what is seen.	Glutathione and lysine, Super oxide dismutase, Vitamin B, B_2, B_6, C, D, selenium, zinc.	Citrus fruits, green peppers, white fish, legumes, cantaloupe, dark green veggies, sprouts, eggs, vegetables, oils, sunlight.
Ciliary Muscle	Attached via ligaments to the lens. Helps with the focusing for close viewing.	Facility and stamina in dealing with change, perspective and space.	Chromium.	Sesame oil, whole grains, cereals. Avoid sugar.
Vitreous	Jelly medium in between retina and lens. Supports the retina and lens.	Stability, sensitivity, and solidity.	Protein supplement, selenium, Vitamin A (Beta Carotene), Vitamin B-complex, C, E, and zinc.	Fresh fruits and vegetables, carrots, yams, cantaloupe.
Retina	Back of the eye—like a satellite dish. Receives the light.	Expansive seeing—receptivity and dealing with the blur and darker side.	Vitamins A, D, C, B, E, zinc, calcium, magnesium, super oxide dismutase.	Fish liver oil, milk, brewers yeast, seafood, soybeans, spinach, sunflower seeds, mushrooms, sunlight
Fovea	Small depression in the retina where 20/20 occurs.	Point of center-alignment with life.	Vitamin B-complex, B_6, B_2, B_3	Vegetables, whole grains, green leafy vegetables, nuts, blackstrap molasses, legumes, seafood, sunflower seeds.
Optic Nerve	Brings blood and nerve supply from the brain.	Movement and flow.	Vitamins B-complex, A, C, D, E	Include live foods such as alfalfa sprouts and other sprouted grains or seeds.
Sclera	White of the eye. Supports and holds the other structures in place.	Rigidity.	Zinc, selenium, calcium, magnesium. Avoid caffeine.	Almonds, figs, greens, beets, grains, sesame and pumpkin seeds, broccoli, asparagus, lentils, garlic, mushrooms, wheat germ, sea vegetables (arame, hiziki, kombu, nori, wakame).
Extraocular Muscles	Six big muscles attached to the sclera.	Tension.	Avoid caffeine, tobacco, alcohol, and especially anti-infection drugs.	Eyebright herb, gotu kola, burdock, comfrey, dandelion, chapparal, echinacea, rosehips.

physician's urging she also decided to have the surgery. After the surgery, the patient continued Integrated Vision Therapy to speed along the healing of her eyes.

Therapeutic Eating

Begin to eat fresh fruits and vegetables, preferably from organic sources. You want to maximize the nutritional value by using produce that has not been sprayed with insecticides or received excess chemical residues in the soils. For better food combining, eat your fruit at different times than your starches. Cut back on eating animal protein, and substitute with soy products such as tofu or tempeh. Eat rice derivatives like rice pasta, and experiment with other grains like quinoa (pronounced "keenwa"), spelt, and kamut. Eating well keeps your body—including your eyes—healthy.

During this therapeutic phase of self-healing, it is best to eliminate all caffeine, tobacco, white flour products, and sugar. It is also advisable to either cut back or eliminate all dairy-derived foods during this phase. Consider using sea vegetables (seaweeds) such as arame, hijiki, nori, wakame, or kombu, because of their rich mineral content. By following this basic nutrition program, most eye conditions respond with functional improvements in vision. You can increase your intake of vitamins and minerals by implementing a general vitamin program, using specific nutrients for each eye condition as shown in table 2. The resources list at the back of this book can also help you to locate holistic practitioners in your area who can assist you.

Imagery and Visualizing

Begin visualizing your eyes becoming healthier no matter how bad you may think your eye condition is. It is important to imagine wellness in the parts of your eyes afflicted by disease. These parts are crying out for attention and love.

Recently, a man consulted me regarding his glaucoma. His idea of developing power behind his eyes was taking extra vitamin C and hoping the pressure would come down. I kept asking him throughout the consultation: "What are your eyes trying to tell you?" When he left my office, this question was firmly planted in his consciousness.

I thought I would never see him again. About two months later, he phoned and said that the condition was now severe enough that his physician had ordered surgery. My patient did not want to undergo this surgical procedure and returned to see me saying he was ready to look deeper into his message to lower the pressure and change his life.

Our next consultation revolved around examining the pressure he puts on himself. He took home a self-healing audiotape of images and specific healing statements. After one month, he lowered the pressure in his eyes to avoid having the surgery. He will need to continue this healing process for a long time, at least until he has mastered the lifestyle application of the learning. He has to learn to live in a different way—lighten up, work less, and rediscover his sense of humor.

Color and Light

One of the most powerful healing forces we have at our disposal is the sun and the full-spectrum of white light that shines down on us. Each color emerges from the white light, affecting every cell in our body. The eyes also need different color frequencies for their sustained function. Try to spend time outdoors in full-spectrum light with your naked eyes exposed for twenty to sixty minutes each day. It is best to do this before ten in the morning or after four in the afternoon, but of course the intensity of the sunlight also depends on the part of the world in which you live. In the Northern Hemisphere, especially in Canada, the sun can be enjoyed all day throughout the winter months, because it is low in the sky and not very intense.

Whenever you have a spare moment, practice "breathing color" into your eyes. Select a specific color from the spectrum: violet, blue, green, yellow, orange, red. Violet is a deep relaxant that can be used to melt tension. Blue is a mild relaxant. Green is a balancing color that can be used to visualize harmony and peace. Yellow is a mild stimulant used to awaken parts of the eye's function. Orange is a slightly stronger stimulant used in the same way as yellow. Red is the strongest stimulant that can be used to visualize healing of tissue, flow of blood, and activating function of the eye. Colors that are adjacent on the color wheel can also be combined, as yellow/green, blue/green, yellow/orange, and red/violet. Imagine the color dancing in your mind, or better still, use gelatin filters such as are used in theater lighting, through which you can look for short ten-minute periods. Once you can see the desired color in your mind, visualize that you are breathing it into your eye, and direct the color to the specific parts of the eye that you wish to heal. If you focus your full, relaxed attention on a specific part of your eye, that structure becomes fully awakened. Feel wellness returning to your eyes. Your eyes will love the attention.

Take your outstretched fingers and slowly wave them in front of your eyes to duplicate the effect of a flashing light. Moving your fingers creates the presence and then the absence of light reaching the eye, as though you were switching lights on and off. Recall that your awareness of your feelings is similarly "on" or "off." Allow the light used in this manner to enliven your inspiration, your spiritual unfolding, by thinking of the light beam as a flashlight that shines on many aspects of your self simultaneously.

The "Short-Arm" Syndrome—
I Am Becoming Wise!

There comes a time when most of us begin experiencing the frustration of trying to thread a needle, determine what delicious meals are on the menu, or read the small print on a package in the supermarket. At first we can overcome the difficulty of reading small print by moving the object further away. Eventually a time comes when our arms definitely seem too short. The good news is that simple nonprescription glasses such as those available at the drugstore can usually alleviate the problem. It is certainly better than getting an arm transplant.

In our younger days, we did not even have to think about focusing and could accomplish seeing the finest of details. But midlife is the age of becoming wise, and focusing clearly becomes the accompanying lesson. We are called upon to pay more attention to being flexible in our dealings with time and space. Our immediate space becomes more precious, and we find ourselves seeking time alone to become clear about what is important for us as individuals. Perhaps this inward searching is the discovery of the spirit within. I have noticed that quite often my patients in their forties begin new careers, focus on redefining their relationships, and claim independence from the strong control of their parents.

In the context of Integrated Vision Therapy, the short-arm syndrome is a time of discovery of self. When my patients understand this, I teach them how to become more focused in their close or near vision. First, begin wearing a weaker lens prescription. In its simplest form, this kind of farsightedness is managed by wearing a reading-lens prescription called a plus lens. You will notice that the reading lenses in the drugstore have little numbers on the tag. The range is usually +1.00 to +3.00. The lower the number, the weaker the lens power.

Find the weakest lens power that lets you see the smallest print possible at about arm's distance. Then begin training yourself to focus more efficiently. Thereafter you can obtain an even weaker lens prescription. Eventually you will notice smaller and smaller details without eyeglasses. This just takes practice, discipline, and the development of new habits of looking and seeing.

Pick up any page with small print and choose a place where you can focus on the white paper and not on the black letters. Begin breathing in and out, paying more attention to the in-breath and the space between the exhale and inhale. Do this for five breaths to refamiliarize yourself with the

**Breathing
and
Tromboning**

act of breathing and seeing more clearly. Now, while taking a small in-breath, move the letters and white background toward your eyes, remembering to focus on the "nothingness" of the white background. Repeat this procedure five times and then look at the letters and notice if they appear any clearer. This vision game is known as "tromboning" and is very effective in stimulating the eye's focusing muscle into action. You may find yourself needing your focusing lenses less as you focus your internal power outward. Enjoy this newly discovered control of your own power.

Lighting

Whenever possible, increase the lighting in your workspace and reading areas of your home. Light causes a constriction of the pupil, resulting in sharper focusing. Spend time outdoors exposing your closed eyes to natural light. Take breaks from your work and shine a reading-lamp light onto your closed eyes. Feel the warmth and imagine you are lying under a tropical sun, soaking up the healing rays.

Whenever your eyes give you the feedback of blurry vision, take a break and palm your eyes. This relaxation of the mind and your eyes will, in most cases, result in clearer vision when you once again look at your reading material.

Help For Your Children's Vision

Over the years, vision therapy optometrists have noticed a sharp increase in the number of children needing eyeglasses. The eyes of our young ones are clearly communicating something very important. The worst possible thing that parents can do is succumb to the limiting belief that traditional compensating lenses for 20/20 vision are going to solve their child's problems. If anything, compensating lenses are going to become addictive, and you and your child will not benefit from what the eye is really communicating. All a compensating lens does is eliminate the symptom of blurred or strained vision, at least for a while, but it does not cure the underlying problem.

Vision therapy optometrists do prescribe what are called stress-relieving or developmental lenses, which in ideal situations and with the accompanying vision-training support guide the brain to make healthier vision choices that will show up in the eye measurements. In some cases, the need for compensating lenses is then reduced. With children the task of retraining their vision is much easier because their visual development is still flexible and malleable. The main point is that, no matter what lens is used, the patient needs to become involved in the process of rehabilitation.

Once your child has been told that he or she needs to wear eyeglasses, consider getting a second opinion. Better still, consult with a vision therapy optometrist and find out what techniques you can learn to initiate your child's healing. Your goal will be to help your child avoid wearing strong, crippling, compensating lenses. Before your child starts to wear glasses, consider a vision therapy program to enhance his or her natural vision skills. This can also prevent vision problems from developing. Here is a basic prevention and maintenance program of vision training that you can easily teach to your child:

Prevention and Maintenance

- Palm your eyes every fifteen minutes, for five to ten breaths.
- While outdoors, close your eyes and let the sunshine beam down onto your eyelids for ten to twenty breaths.
- Every fifteen minutes, focus your eyes and attention on a poster or picture in the distance. This is particularly good if the child is reading, watching TV, or playing video games.
- Practice crossing your eyes. Eye crossing is fun, and it is a very powerful vision-enhancer. Your child should be able to notice two objects in the distance when he or she is in the eye-crossing mode. Do the exercises along with your child—you will benefit, too.

Parents often feel alarmed and helpless when told their child needs eye surgery. Surgical procedures are, by and large, mainly cosmetic in the case of crossed or wandering eyes. It may seem reasonable to believe that if the eyes are straight after a surgical procedure, then the vision through each eye is working well and integrating in the brain. At best, this only happens 30 percent of the time—it is also not unusual that the surgical procedure must be repeated at a later date. Another frequent occurrence is that an opposite condition develops after time: for example, if surgery was performed to straighten a crossed eye, a wandering eye condition may later result.

Surgery

If you have been told that your child needs eye surgery, the first thing to do is to obtain a second opinion, again preferably with a vision therapy optometrist. At least consider a program of vision therapy in which two-eyed vision can be retrained in its own time. Your family may learn some very important information about the dynamics of your relationships; I frequently find that a family situation is contributing to the child's eye condition. When I assist a child or young adult, I very often involve the parents in the training as well.

Learning "Problems"

According to Gary Bachara and optometrist Joel Zaba, between 16 and 20 percent of the school population have difficulty learning to read and keeping up with the other children within the traditional curriculum models of teaching. The clinical research published in optometric and educational journals suggests strong relationships between vision perception, two-eyed skills, learning to read, and maintaining high levels of comprehension. Surprisingly, these children typically have 20/20 eyesight. The danger is that some more traditional optometrists might say that if the child can see 20/20, his eyes are fine and that vision, therefore, has no bearing on the child's difficulty with reading. As a parent, you can become very confused with these differing professional opinions. My suggestion is again that you consult with a well-respected vision therapy optometrist in your area.

Ask friends for an eye doctor they can recommend, and make a decision that matches your personal philosophy of life. My experience and choice is to incorporate complementary processes wherever possible. The new school of integrated vision therapists is comprised of individuals who have taken a step beyond traditional optometry. They have undertaken personal growth themselves, and that makes them even more sensitive to your child's special vision needs.

Because vision follows a developmental path, encourage eye and hand activities appropriate for your child's age. Involve her in physical movement and ball games. Better still, let your child bounce on a medium-sized trampoline and engage her mind in spelling and arithmetic manipulations while bouncing. A brightly colored hanging ball, attached by a string, can be a wonderful toy.

Have the child hit the ball with alternate hands while calling out shapes, colors, or names of fruits or vegetables. Following the ball with her eyes teaches the child how to integrate the two hemispheres of the brain. You can observe the effectiveness of this by seeing if the child's eyes move symmetrically together. If not, cover the preferred eye and repeat the game. Remember, if your child becomes bored or seems unable to perform the activity, have her palm the eyes for five breaths. This relaxation gives the child a chance to recover some visual focus.

Living
Your Daily Vision

Our deeper understanding tells us that a truly evolved being is one that values others more than itself, and values love more than it values the physical world and what is in it.

—Gary Zukav

Y ou have come a long way in taking charge of your vision. You understand that vision is more than the physical functioning of your eyes. You now know you can take charge of your life and create the vision you desire. Reread the notes you made from previous chapters. What steps do you intend to take to implement your program?

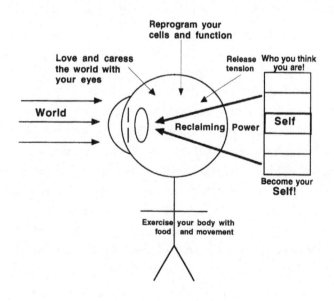

RECLAIMING
YOUR POWER:
HOW YOU SEE

When you visit your eye doctor, you are now going to be empowered by participating as a partner. Your new knowledge and broader experience of what makes your vision clear will assist you in asking your optometrist for what you need and want. So many of us nibble at the menu of vision, thinking that the only choices available are what traditional optometry and ophthalmology can offer. Integrated Vision Therapy has opened up wider doors for you, allowing new perceptions to blossom.

Every moment of life becomes a therapeutic opportunity to generate new visions. Being in my kitchen at home can be an experience of great creativity for me. Looking in the refrigerator and imagining a meal is as useful a practice of vision as shifting my eyes or looking at an Eye-C chart. Washing a bunch of carrots freshly picked from the garden is also such an exercise. Your vision journey is like the preparation of a meal in the kitchen. You search out the insightful ingredients you will need, spice them with some imagination, and let it all simmer for a while. Then you present your creation to the world, to be slowly savored.

Bringing health and clarity to your eyes requires planning your vision menu with imagination. What stimulates your individual imagination? At a photographic shoot on the island of Molokai in the Hawaiian island chain, about fifteen of us photographed a magnificent sunset with a grove of palm trees silhouetted in the foreground. Two days later we had a group showing of our slides. Even though we had all photographed the same scene, our slides were amazingly unique. Each of our individual imaginations created a slightly different vision of how we saw this spectacle. I enjoyed the way others saw what I didn't see. This example of how many possible perceptions are available to sculpt the individual view of life motivated me to expand the possible ways of appreciating what my eyes can allow me to see.

Patty

Patty was seventy years young when she first visited me. She wore bifocals primarily for reading. A friend suggested she see me for symptoms of double vision and confusion. Patty had been widowed; shortly thereafter she developed an aneurysm in the brain, which put her in a coma for four weeks and left her with high blood pressure. Patty described her vision through the left eye as "wonky." The eye wandered outward, and testing of the retina and macula (with dye) indicated very little usable vision. The retina was not being used much, and macular deterioration had begun.

Patty covered her left eye when she read in order to eliminate the double vision. Her Harry perceiving side was perfect. Patty appeared to be an emotionally strong woman. In spite of the double vision, for which she also used a compensating prism lens, she was driving and playing golf.

How could I guide Patty in discovering insight from her eye condition? I first had her cover her right eye, and slowly introduced her to looking through Sally. I was surprised at how little she could see through her left eye. She didn't feel much emotionally.

Within a few months, her perceptions through her left eye began to awaken. Integrated Vision Therapy progressed, Patty mentioned her late husband. She talked about him as if he were still present. Even when Patty bought a new car, she told me that she asked him how he felt about the purchase. I began to suspect that her left-eye condition was related to Patty's holding on to her past. I didn't believe she had fully accepted her husband's departure. Patty denied the grief she felt at the time, instead taking on a tough-male persona. She could manage. She would keep a stiff upper lip and not let her husband's death affect her. Patty's buried feelings may have contributed to the destruction of the retina and of macular tissue. She continued her life as if nothing serious had happened, keeping busy to avoid the reality of her eye condition and her new life without her partner.

As we worked together, Patty's interest in her health intensified. She began volunteering to help people who were dying of debilitating diseases. Patty began playing golf without her eyeglasses and gave up wearing the prism lens that had been compensating for her double vision.

She continued to drive effortlessly in spite of the double vision. "I feel much more comfortable with the second image now. I know where it is," Patty commented at one of our sessions. I waited until the seventh month of her Integrated Vision Therapy program before I raised the question of her secret purpose. I had Patty lie down and flashed red lights into her left eye. The color red is a powerful stimulant and activates blood flow and tissue regeneration. Red can evoke emotions of anger, denial, and frustration. Patty was using integrated breathing and was quite relaxed. I began talking to her in a very quiet voice.

"It seems that the disease condition of your left eye has to do with fully acknowledging the living and dying aspects of your life. It is time for you to face your perceptions of the completion of death and the beginning of life. What does this mean to you? Your eye condition is your opportunity to wake up to some other aspects of your life now and in the future. Consider your life in the future and how you feel about dying. Keep looking at your life in the past, today, and what you would like for the future. How does your eye condition serve to wake you up to some other possibilities for your life? As you wake up the old perceptions through your left eye, explore how you wish to see your life through renewed vision. Could some secret purpose for living now emerge that is different from the past? Do you need to let go of old perceptions to make room for deeper feelings to guide you in transforming your vision of what you are to achieve for your remaining days? How do you feel about dying? By living a life aligned with your purpose, can you produce a death process that is peaceful and free of pain? Your eye disease is signaling an awakening of your spirit. This means facing your true perceptions of a merged soul and personality. The aware-ness that accrues is for both the living and the dying parts of your life. Align-ing with your purpose and living in your vision better prepares you for dying. You are preparing for the continuation of your soul's journey. Keep looking at the edge you gain as your eye becomes healthy."

Patty continued to breathe, and I suggested that as she felt her blood flow into her left eye carrying healthy nutrients, perhaps her life would flow more freely. I had her consider that the light entering her eye was allowing increased blood flow and regeneration, and this was simultaneously con-nected to some greater flow of change to all people on Earth. Taking charge of her left eye was stimulating intuitive processes of what has been called the "collective consciousness" of all our planet's inhabitants. As Patty de-veloped her feeling, emotional qualities, she was contributing to a change in all those people with whom she interacted. As she learned to receive more in life, she would be activating this aspect in others. Perhaps Patty would attract love back into her life.

As the effects of the Integrated Vision Therapy settled in, Patty began to feel different. "I listen more to people. This is not something I used to do. I would blank people out," she informed me. Her left-eye vision began to get sharper, losing its fuzzy edges. Patty began to wean herself from her sunglasses. The colored light she was learning to receive through her left eye had programmed her brain to let light in more effectively. This resulted in her being able to feel more. The emotional correlate of the frequency of the red light shining into the left eye had been successfully integrated into her conscious awareness. This specific frequency of light had opened up that part of Patty's emotions, making it possible for her to see her purpose.

Betty

At age twenty-four, Betty had been diagnosed with a disease condition of the retina and the choroid (structure underneath the retina) of the left eye. This resulted in a loss of her central foveal sight, her looking as well as her field of vision. A prominent professor of ophthalmology in England stated her prognosis was uncertain, although a spontaneous recovery was possible.

When I first met her, two years after the diagnosis, a recovery had not yet occurred. As in many disease situations, Betty had a high degree of nearsightedness. She was overweight, but proudly announced that she had cut back her cigarette smoking to two packs a week. Prior to the onset of her left-eye vision loss, Betty had been plagued by severe headaches. She would wake up with them and never left home without her painkillers. Betty was a pianist and teacher. She reported that after a performance, her headaches became worse. Her piano rehearsals were her addiction. "I avoid reality by rehearsing," she candidly admitted at our first visit.

My first approach in providing Integrated Vision Therapy was to patch her right eye. She needed to fully submerge herself in the experience of once again seeing through the left eye. Her functional vision through this eye was negligible when we began therapy.

When I directed a bright, red light into her left eye, she could only distinguish the redness to the right. She felt very vulnerable with the patch on. "This is not a role I'm comfortable with," she said. Betty suddenly recalled a visit she had made to a doctor of Chinese medicine in England, who informed her of the relationship between the health of her liver and her eye condition. He described her liver as being dry and thirsty. He immediately took her off the corticosteroids that another doctor had prescribed, and used Chinese herbs to restore balance to the liver. For thousands of years the Chinese have known that the functioning of the liver follows the same acupuncture meridians as the eyes. If the liver is malfunctioning, the eyes' ability to function is affected. Also, according to Traditional Chinese Medicine the liver is the seat of anger. If anger is discharged, health improves and the eyes will have a brighter, clearer appearance.

Betty described herself as having been a tomboy in her childhood. The connection between her perceptions of being a tomboy correlated to the dominance of her vision through Harry, the more male oriented behavior. Betty had had a difficult childhood. Her mother, Anne, had cancer of the bowel and an irritated colon. She was a workaholic; it was a struggle to get her to slow down. Betty described Anne as feeling unloved. This was played out in Betty's childhood: Betty felt choked and suffocated by her mother, who needed to possess and control. While Betty was wearing the patch a headache began, and Betty related that her mother was a headache.

I was curious to look at the colored parts of the iris, wondering if there were any structural patterns related to her retinal condition that may have been genealogically carried down from her mother's side of the family. As is the case in many patients, Betty had a large brown spot in the four-o'clock position of the left eye. According to the Rayid method of iris interpretation, unresolved anger was present in the maternal family tree. Since her mother had not effectively dealt with this anger tendency, Betty had to choose between acting out her anger or developing a passion toward something in her life. She was clearer and more dominant through her right eye.

On Betty's second visit, I covered her right eye and asked her to describe what she could see. She described how, when she was in the presence of artificial light, she seemed to retain an afterimage of the light of the situation. She had been patching quite often during the past month, and the only vision she had through the left eye was grayish and cloudy. As I directed a red flashing-light source into her left eye, Betty was able to identify points of light off to the right side. I continued this procedure while asking her questions in a quiet voice. As the vision therapy took effect, I encouraged Betty to talk about her feelings. Tears began to fall and she reported feeling sad.

The four years prior to the loss of her left-eye vision had been a period of obsessive work. Betty had run away from emotional problems with friends. She had been very close to a woman named Frances. Betty's roommate at the time became insanely jealous of her friendship with Frances. When Frances got together with a man, Betty ended up with neither woman's friendship. She described this time as the time she "put the lid on strong." Betty became very sick and had a "miniature nervous breakdown" just prior to the time her eyesight began to fail. She continued: "Those three years were miserable. I went inside, didn't take on any more work, and hated being with myself. I was a very unhappy person."

I then had Betty jump up and down on a trampoline while she called out numbers on each bounce, from one to ten, forward and then backward. I added new instructions as she became more proficient. First, Betty had to clap her hands on five and say the number. Then she substituted the number eight with the word "Mom," keeping the clap on five. This progressed until she reached her threshold and witnessed herself trying to cover up for confusion and loss of memory. I seized the opportunity to coach her on how to stay present, trust her memory, and get into the flow. Her biggest challenge was learning how to see in her mind by visualizing the instructional sequence rather than memorizing it. Then I had her practice her physical balance in a new way, by again patching her right eye.

Once she mastered the sequence and was able to transfer the learning and experience, I had her rest and stimulated her left eye with the flashing red light. The frequency of the flashes matched the brainwave pattern known as alpha rhythm, at about eight to thirteen cycles per second. This frequency enhances the brightness of light as it strikes the retina and then stimulates the optic nerve pathway to the brain. This was particularly important because she felt as if she were having a nervous breakdown.

Betty relaxed and began to rephrase her perceptions about the difficult phase of her life. This included a new relationship between Betty and light. When we experience disease, we are less able to take in light. Sunlight will create an allergic reaction, usually in the form of oversensitivity. Betty had been wearing sunglasses most days, but now she said, "I know how positive the sun is, and it is not the enemy." She continued: "Time has passed

. . . I have let go of something . . . I don't need the drug of addictive relationships . . . I just need to be loved!" These statements demonstrate the emergence of the power that would ignite the healing of her Sally retina.

Betty needed to shift her former negative perceptions for her eyes to function in a healthy and clear way. Her purpose was clear—she wanted to play the piano, perform, and teach. Her way of expressing this vision, however, was out of balance. The secret for Betty was to maintain harmony within her hectic lifestyle.

Betty's face beamed with a youthful glow when she left. Her parting words represented the shift in her perceptions. "I wouldn't be where I am now if that unpleasant experience and eye condition hadn't happened."

The Tibetan tradition emphasizes that no matter how many exercises keep you busy in your life, they won't help unless you are totally committed to having clarity. One of my patients used a ritual to set her sights on clearer vision: "When I burned my eyeglasses, I had to leave my old perceptions behind and develop new ones," she said. "I had to *feel* in order to *see*."

How do you clear your mind and begin to feel? Remember the relaxation steps outlined earlier. Spend time in nature. Relax in your favorite chair. Have a massage or a foot rub. Exercise or move on a trampoline. Soak in a hot tub or relax in a sauna. Do you remember Sam, who so wanted to be accepted into the police academy? He needed to open up his emotional side more. I suggested that he talk to his mother and find out more about his birth. He gave me a puzzled look and said: "That is definitely hot-tub material!" For him, exploring previous addictive relationships with his blurry left eye was to be done in the hot tub. The Buddhist monks find mindfulness through silent contemplation; the painter embellishes his canvas with images; the businessperson makes new deals. For you, clearing your mind might be accomplished during gardening, fishing, telling stories to children, or talking to older people. During those times you are in observation of yourself. You are mindful.

The challenge to be clear puts the burden on you. You must be responsible for every perception and action you observe. If you lapse into visual unconsciousness for one moment, you lessen your power as a human being. Tell your optometrist you wish to *participate* in your visual well-being. Dentists have taught us to take care of our teeth between office visits. Sharper vision can be achieved by using the Eye-C charts and weaker lens prescriptions, speaking positively, patching, palming, nose crossing and eye crossing, yawning, and integrated breathing while watching a candle flame. Through language you can voice your clear desires and intention. Sharp vision needs an active soul. How do you intend to apply yourself?

For most of your life, you have made choices influenced by others. It is time to break your habits. Zajonc says, "The habits of our culture, the dogmas of our education, constrain our sight." We are so busy rushing around most of the time that we miss those special soul moments. What habits do you still hold onto that restrict your ability to conjure up fresh perceptions? Get to know your body. The practice of yoga, for example, can sharpen your perceptions so you can feel the restrictions of your body. Body tightness and stress are quite often related to visual limitations. Through yoga and other forms of exercise, you can learn about your points of resistance. As one Tibetan teacher says, "Go into the pain!" You don't have to feel pain in your eyes in order to get clarity. Find your secret purpose. Stretch yourself to your limits. Negotiate your blur, and see the letters on the Eye-C chart begin popping into focus. Soon you will have perfect 20/20 vision through your weaker prescription, then you can return to your optometrist for the next reduction.

Ancient ritual could become useful at this stage of your process. My patients Rosanne and Lorna used ceremonies as a way to let go of their past perceptions and addictive need for their glasses. When she was ready to move to a weaker lens prescription, Rosanne went to the ocean and, standing on a dock, ceremoniously threw her glasses into the water. Her glasses were like a hook to the past, and the process enabled her to embark on her new life and vision. Lorna decided to use the hot energy of a fire to burn her glasses. Watching her stylish $600 Silhouette frame and lenses burn, she made a commitment to begin a new way of looking and seeing.

One Last Example

I heard of a physician who was bored with practicing medicine. His passion in life was camping outdoors. He decided to close his practice and pursue his soul purpose. He found a camping-equipment company that needed to have its gear tested. He became the company's consultant and now spends his time traveling, hiking, and camping. You may run into him one day while hiking in the Colorado mountains.

Appendix

The Essential Integrated Vision Therapy Program

Page references to this text are given for each component of the program.

Weaker lens prescription: 71, 73

Identifying iris type: 23

Visualizing the anatomy: 134–138

Vision exercises

    Naked vision: 142, 146

    Far and near Eye-C charts: 51, 52, 64, 93–94

    Single/double candle watching: 55–58

    Nose and eye crossing: 55–58

    Eye uncrossing: 57–58

    Patching: 71–72, 120–121

    Multidimensional picture: 58–59

    Astigmatism fusion games: 144–146

Journal exercises

    Identifying incompletions: 116, 120

    What I want is: 66

    The way I am likely to sabotage myself is: 66

    Identifying past visually related events: 114–115, 132

Relaxation exercises

    Integrated breathing: 36–37

    Palming: 100, 120

    Relaxation narrative: 134–138

    Stillness: 93–94

Creative visualization techniques: 63–64, 93–94, 125

Empowering through language: 100–101

Twenty-one-day program—summary: 128
    Therapeutic eating: 33–34, 155
    Color and light: 156, 158
    Tromboning: 158
    Movement (trampoline): 76–77
    Light (sun or full-spectrum light bulb): 46, 158
    Finger-waving in front of the eyes: 156–157

Bibliography

Suggested Reading

Ackerman, D. *A Natural History of the Senses*. New York: Random House, 1991.

Bates, W. H. *The Bates Method for Better Eyesight Without Glasses*. New York: Jove/Harcourt Brace Jovanovich, 1978.

Berendt, J.E. *The Third Ear: On Listening to the World*. Dorset, England: Element Books, 1988.

Berger, J. *Ways of Seeing*. New York: Penguin Books, 1972.

Berne, S. *Creating Your Personal Vision*. Santa Fe, N.M.: Color Stone Press, 1994.

Bowers, K. S. *Hypnosis for the Seriously Curious*. New York: Jason Aronson, Inc., 1977.

Brennan, B. A. *Hands of Light: A Guide to Healing through the Human Energy Field*. New York: Bantam Books, 1987.

Bryant, D. *The Kin of Ata Are Waiting for You*. New York: Random House, 1971.

Burroughs, S. *Healing for the Age of Enlightenment*. Auburn, Calif.: Self-published, 1976.

Chodron, P. *Open Heart, Clear Mind*. Ithaca, N.Y.: Snow Lion Publications, 1990.

Chopra, D. *Ageless Body, Timeless Mind: The Quantum Alternative to Growing Old*. New York: Harmony, 1993.

———. *Return of the Rishi: A Doctor's Story of Spiritual Transformation and Ayurvedic Healing*. Boston: Houghton Mifflin Company, 1988.

Csikszentmihalyi, M. *Flow: The Psychology of Optimal Experience*. New York: Harper Perennial, 1990.

DeRohan, C. *Right Use of Will: Healing and Evolving the Emotional Body*. Santa Fe, N.M.: Four Winds Publications, 1984.

Dominguez, J., and V. Robin, *Your Money or Your Life*. New York: Penguin, 1992.

Donahue, P. *The Human Animal*. New York: Simon and Schuster, 1985.

Epstein, G. *Healing Visualizations: Creating Health Through Imagery*. New York: Bantam Books, 1989.

Exeter, M. *Living at the Heart of Creation: Practical Wisdom for Extraordinary Times*. Loveland, Colo.: Foundation House Publications, 1990.

Forrest, E. B. *Stress and Vision*. Santa Ana, Calif.: Optometric Extension Program Foundation, 1988.

Franck, F. *The Zen of Seeing*. New York: Vintage Books, 1973.

Gimbel, T. *Form, Sound, Colour and Healing*. Essex, England: The C.W. Daniel Company Limited, 1987.

Goodrich, J. *Natural Vision Improvement*. Berkeley, Calif.: Celestial Arts, 1985.

Greenwood, M., and P. Nunn. *Paradox and Healing: Medicine, Mythology and Transformation*. Victoria, B.C., Canada: Meridian House, 1992.

Gregory, R. L. *Eye and Brain: The Psychology of Seeing*. London: World University Library, 1969.

Gyaltsen, S. T. *Heart Drops of Dharmakaya*. New York: Snow Lion Publications, 1993.

Harrison, J. *Love Your Disease: It's Keeping You Healthy!* Norta Ride, N.S.W., Australia: Angus & Robertson, 1984.

Hendricks, G., and K. Hendricks. *Centering and the Art of Intimacy*. New Jersey: Prentice-Hall, Inc, 1985.

Hetzel, R. *The New Physician: Tapping the Potential for True Health*. Wantima South, Victoria, Australia: Houghton Mifflin, 1991.

Hoffman, H. S. *Vision and the Art of Drawing*. Englewood Cliffs, N.J.: Prentice-Hall, Inc, 1989.

Huxley, A. *The Art of Seeing*. Seattle: Montana Books, 1975.

Jampolsky, G.G. *Love Is Letting Go of Fear*. New York: Bantam Books, 1970.

Jeffers, S. *Feel The Fear and Do It Anyway*. New York: Fawcett, 1987.

Johnson, D. *What the Eye Reveals: An Introduction to the Rayid Method of Iris Interpretation*. Goleta, Calif.: Rayid Publications, 1984.

Joudry, P. *Sound Therapy for the Walk Man*. Dalmeny, Sask., Canada: Steele and Steele, 1989.

Kaplan, R. M. *Seeing Without Glasses* (formerly *Seeing Beyond 20/20*). Hillsboro, Oreg.: Beyond Words, 1994.

Keleman, S. *Emotional Anatomy*. Berkeley, CA.: Center Press, 1985.

Krieger, D. *The Therapeutic Touch: How to Use Your Hands to Help or to Heal*. Englewood Cliffs, N.J.: Prentice-Hall, Inc. 1979.

Kushi, M. *Natural Healing through Macrobiotics.* Tokyo: Japan Publications, Inc. 1978.

Laborde, G. Z. *Influencing with Integrity: Management Skills For Communication and Negotiation.* Palo Alto, Calif.: Syntony Inc. Publishing Co., 1984.

Lad, V. *Ayurveda: The Science of Self-Healing.* Santa Fe, N.M.: Lotus Press, 1984.

Leviton, R. *Seven Steps to Better Vision.* Brookline, Mass.: East West/Natural Health Books, 1992.

Liberman, J. *Take Off Your Glasses and See: How to Heal Your Eyesight and Expand Your Insight.* New York: Crown Publishers, 1995.

Liberman, J. *Light Medicine of the Future.* Santa Fe, N.M.: Bear & Company, 1991.

Liedloff, J. *The Continuum Concept: Allowing Human Nature to Work Successfully.* New York: Addison-Wesley, 1977.

Long, M. E. "The Sense of Sight." *National Geographic* 3, no. 41, 1992.

Lusseyran, J. *And There Was Light.* New York: Parabola Books, 1988.

Marshall, E. *Eye Language: Understanding the Eloquent Eye.* New York: New Trend, 1983.

Melina, V., B. David, and V. Harrison. *Becoming Vegetarian: The Complete Guide to Adopting a Healthy Vegetarian Diet.* Toronto: Macmillan Canada, 1994.

Mendelsohn, R. S. *How to Raise a Healthy Child . . . In Spite of Your Doctor.* New York: Ballantine Books, 1984.

Millman, D. *Way of the Peaceful Warrior: A Book That Changes Lives.* Tiburon, Calif.: H. J. Kramer, Inc., 1984.

Mindell, A. *Working with the Dreaming Body.* Boston: Routledge & Kegan Paul, 1985.

Mindell, A., and A. Mindell. *Riding the Horse Backwards: Process Work in Theory and Practice.* London: Penguin, 1992.

Morningstar, A., and V. Desai. *The Ayurvedic Cookbook: A Personalized Guide to Good Nutrition and Health.* Wilmot, Wis.: Lotus Light, 1990.

N. E. Thing Enterprises. *Magic Eye: A New Way of Looking at the World.* Kansas City: Andrews and McMell, 1993.

Ohashi, W. *Do-It-Yourself Shiatsu: How to Perform the Ancient Japanese Art of Acupuncture without Needles.* New York: E. P. Dutton, 1976.

Ornish, D. *Program for Reversing Heart Disease.* New York: Random House, 1990.

Padus, E., and the editors of *Prevention Magazine. The Complete Guide to Your Emotions and Your Health.* Emmaus, Penn.: Rodale Press, 1986.

Patterson, F. *Photography and the Art of Seeing.* Toronto: Key Porter Books, 1985.

Pearce, J. C. *Evolution's End.* San Francisco: HarperSanFrancisco, 1992.

Rinpoche, S. *The Tibetan Book of Living and Dying.* New York: Harper-Collins, 1992.

Rotte, J., and K. Yamamoto. *Vision: A Holistic Guide to Healing the Eyesight.* New York: Japan Publications, 1986.

Schaef, A. W. *When Society Becomes an Addict.* New York: Harper & Row, 1987.

Schneider, M. *Self Healing: My Life and Vision.* New York: Routledge & Kegan Paul Inc, 1987.

Schwarz, J. *Human Energy Systems.* New York: E. P. Dutton, 1980.

Seiderman, A. S., and S. E. Marcus. *20/20 Is Not Enough: The New World of Vision.* New York: Ballantine Books, 1989.

Selby, J. *The Visual Handbook: The Complete Guide to Seeing More Clearly.* Dorset, England: Element Books, 1987.

Selye, H. *Stress without Distress,* New York: J. B. Lippincott, 1974.

Shankman, A. L. *Vision Enhancement Training.* Santa Ana, Calif.: Optometric Extension Program Foundation, 1988.

Trachtman, J. N. *The Etiology of Vision Disorders: A Neuroscience Model.* Santa Ana, Calif.: Optometric Extension Program Foundation, 1990.

Vernon, M. D. *The Psychology of Perception.* Middlesex, England: Penguin, 1962.

Verny, T., and J. Kelly. *The Secret Life of the Unborn Child.* New York: Dell Publishing, 1981.

Von Senden, M. *Space and Sight: The Perception of Space and Shape in the Congenitally Blind Before and After Operation,* Trans. Peter Heath. Glencoe, Ill.: The Free Press, 1960.

Walker, M. *The Power of Color: The Art and Science of Making Colors Work for You.* New York: Avery Publishing Group, 1991.

Wood, B. *The Healing Power of Color: How to Use Color to Improve Your Mental, Physical and Spiritual Well-being.* Rochester, Vt.: Destiny Books, 1992.

Yatri. *Unknown Man: The Mysterious Birth of a New Species.* New York: Simon and Schuster, 1988.

Zajone, A. *Catching the Light: The Entwined History of Light and Mind,* New York: Bantam, 1993.

Zukav, G. *The Seat of the Soul.* New York: Simon & Schuster, 1989.

REFERENCES

Bachara, G. H., J. N. Zaba, and L. M. Raskin. 1975–76. Human figure drawings and LD children. *Academic Therapy* 6(2):217–222.

Bachara, G. H., and J. N. Zaba. 1976. Psychological Affects of Visual Training. *Academic Therapy* 12(1):99–104.

Baker, R. S., and M. M. Steed. 1990. Restoration of function in paralytic strabismus: alternative methods of therapy. *Binocular Vision Quarterly* 5(4):203–211.

Bracewell, R. M., and H. M. Stein. 1990. Specialization of the right hemisphere for visuomotor control. *Neurology* 40:284–292.

Carr, D., T. W. Jackson, and D. J. Madden. 1992. The effect of age on driving skills. *Journal of the American Geriatrics Society.* 40(6):567–73.

Collins, F. L., J. A. Ricci, and J. A. Burkett. 1981. Behavioral training for myopia: long term maintenance of improved acuity. *Behaviour Research and Therapy* 19(3):265–268.

Cool, S. J. 1993. Clinicians should be open-minded and explore the clinical value of new therapies or myth and metaphor, fact and datum in the art and science of clinical care. *Journal of Behavioral Optometry* 4:119–121.

Filatov, V. P., and V. A. Verbitska. 1946. Treatment of retinitis pigmentosa. *American Review of Soviet Medicine* 3:385–480.

Gallop, S. 1994. Myopia reduction. *Journal of Behavioral Optometry* 5(5):115–120.

Goss, D. A., and R. L. Winkler. 1983. Progression of myopia in youth: age of cessation. *American Journal of Optometry and Physiological Optics* 60:651–658.

Greene, P. R. 1980. Mechanical considerations in myopia: relative effects of accommodation, accommodative convergence, intraocular pressure and extra-ocular muscles. *American Journal of Optometry and Physiological Optics* 47:902–914.

Hall, P. S., and B. C. Wick. 1991. The relationship betwen ocular functions and reading achievement. *Journal of Pediatric Ophthalmology and Strabismus* 28:17–19.

Johnson, R., and J. N. Zaba. 1994. The link: vision and illiteracy. *Journal of Behavioral Optometry* 5(2):41.

Kane, M. 1992. Vision therapy: Its impact on intelligence tests. *Journal of Optometric Vision Development* 23:39–41.

Kaplan, R. M. 1976. The interdisciplinary team approach—a case study. *Journal of the American Optometric Association* 47(9):1153–1166.

———. 1976. The intermodality relationship of auditory and vision perception. *Journal of the American Optometric Association* 47:29–32.

———. 1977. A comparison of left and right eye speed of recognition values in average and below readers. *Optometric Extension Program Papers* 30(2).

———. 1977. Orthoptics or surgery? A case report. *Optometric Weekly* 68(39):33–66.

———. 1978. Hypnosis—new horizons for optometry. *Review of Optometry* 115(1):53–58.

———. 1983. Changes in form visual fields in reading disabled children, produced by syntonic (colored light) stimulation. *The International Journal of Biosocial Research* 5(1):20–33.

———. 1994. Beyond 20/20 vision. *Insight: Rayid International Newsletter* 3:6–7.

———. 1994. Enhancing vision with herbs. *Journal of the Canadian Association of Herbal Practitioners* 32(1):5.

Lane, B. C. 1982. Myopia prevention and reversal: new data confirms the interaction of accommodative stress and deficit-inducing nutrition. *Journal of the International Academy of Preventive Medicine* 7(3):17–30.

Ogle, K.N., T.G. Martens, and J.A. Dyer. 1967. *Oculomotor imbalance in binocular vision and fixation disparity*. Philadelphia: Lea and Febiger, 39–73.

Orfield, A. 1994. Seeing space: undergoing brain re-programming to reduce myopia. *Journal of Behavioral Optometry* 5(5):123–131.

Ott, J. N. 1985. Color and light: Their effects on plants, animals and people. *The International Journal of Biosocial Research* 7:1–35.

Passo, M. S., et al. 1991. Exercise training reduces intraocular pressure among subjects suspected of having glaucoma. *Archives of Ophthalmology* 109:1096–1098.

Roscoe, S. N., and D. H. Couchman. 1987. Improving visual performance through volitional focus control. *Human Factors* 29(3):311–325.

Rosen, R. C., H. R. Schiffman, and A. S. Cohen. 1984. Behavior modification and the treatment of myopia. *Behavior Modification* 8(2):131–154.

Rosenfield, M., and B. Gilmartin. 1987. Effect of a near vision task on the response AC/A of a myopic population. *Ophthalmic and Physiological Optics* 7:225–233.

Sakai, T., M. Murata, and T. Amemiya. 1992. Effect of long-term treatment of glaucoma with Vitamin B12. *Glaucoma* 14:167–170.

Shapiro, F. 1989. Eye movement desensitization: a new treatment for post-traumatic stress disorder. *Journal of Behavioral Therapy and Experimental Psychiatry* 20(3):211–217.

———. 1989. Efficacy of the eye movement desensitization procedure in the treatment of traumatic memories. *Journal of Traumatic Stress* 2(2):199–223.

Sherman, A. 1993. Myopia can often be prevented, controlled or eliminated. *Journal of Behavioral Optometry* 4:16.

Shotwell, A. J. 1981. Plus lenses, prisms and bifocal effects on myopia progression in military students. *American Journal of Optometry and Physiological Optics* 58:349–354.

———. 1984. Plus lenses, prism and bifocal effects on myopia progression in military students. Part II. *American Journal of Optometry and Physiological Optics* 61:112–117.

Siderov, J., and L. DiGuglielmo. 1991. Binocular accommodative facility in prepresbyopic adults and its relation to symptoms. *Optometry and Vision Science* 68:49–53.

Sperduto, R. D., D. Seigel, J. Roberts, M. Rowland. 1983. Prevalence of myopia in the United States. *Archives of Ophthalmology* 101:405–407.

Trachtman, J. N., 1987. Biofeedback of accommodation to reduce myopia—a review. *American Journal of Optometry and Physiological Optics* 64(8):639–643.

Trachtman, J., V. Giambalvo, and V. Feldman. 1981. Biofeedback of accommodation to reduce functional myopia. *Biofeedback-Self-Regul.* 6(4): 547–562.

Trachtman, J. and V. Giambalvo. 1991. The Baltimore myopia study 40 years later. *Journal of Behavioral Optometry* 2:47–50.

Velasco e Cruz, A. A. 1990. Historical roots of 20/20 as a (wrong) standard value of normal visual acuity. *Optometric and Vision Science* 67(8):661.

Wiggins, N., and K. Daum. 1991. Visual discomfort and astigmatic refractive errors in VDT use. *Journal of the American Optometric Association* 68:680–684.

Wilson, M. E. J. 1992. Adult amblyopia reversed by contralateral cataract formation. *Pediatric Ophthalmology and Strabismus* 29(2):100–102.

Young, F. A. 1963. The effect of restricted visual space on the refractive error of the young monkey eye. *Investigative Ophthalmology* 2:571–577.

Young, F. A., G. A. Leary, W. R. Baldwin, D. C. West, R. A. Bos, E. Harrie, and C. Johnson. 1969. The transmission of refractive errors within Eskimo families. *Archives of the American Academy of Optometry* 49:676–685.

Zadnick, K., et al. 1994. The effect of parental history of myopia on children's eye size. *Journal of the American Medical Association* 27(17):1323–1327.

Zeki, S. 1992. The visual image in mind and brain. *Scientific American* 267(3):69–76.

Resources

College of Optometrists in Vision Development
www.covd.org
Referral for optometrists who provide vision therapy services.

Optometric Extension Program Foundation Inc.
1921 E. Carnegie Avenue, Suite 3-L
Santa Ana, CA 92705-5811
(714) 250-8070
www.oep.org
Optometrists who could prescribe weaker lens prescriptions.

North America

Dr. Robert-Michael Kaplan
Beyond 20/20 Vision®
P.O. Box 68
Roberts Creek, B.C. V0N 2W0
Canada
Fax: (604) 608-3519
email: robertokap@sunshine.net
www.robertokaplan.com

Europe

Institute Integrative Sehtherapie
Eckpergasse 31/7
A-1180-Wein, Europe
Dr. Kaplan Phone: 0043 676 619 2048
Fax: 0043 22 33 55 436
email: robertokap@sunshine.net
www.robertokaplan.at

Additional programs and services

Although reading this book is one way to improve your seeing potential, I also offer phone and e-mail consultation support to help you achieve your goal of better eyesight. During these consultations, your progress and problematic areas are discussed and solutions are offered for your specific challenges. The consultations are designed to recharge your interest and enthusiasm, as well as provide practical pointers to enhance your vision fitness program by identifying appropriate vision fitness tools for your diagnosed eye condition.

For further information about phone consultations and seminars or to order vision fitness programs, self-healing CDs, pinholes, color balancing kits, or other products, please contact me at:

Dr. Robert-Michael Kaplan
Beyond 20/20 Vision®
P.O. Box 68
Roberts Creek, B.C. V0N 2W0
Canada
Fax: 604-608-3519
e-mail: robertokap@sunshine.net
www.robertokaplan.com

For a referral to a vision therapy Optometrist in your area please visit the Web site www.vision3d.com and click on directory.

I wish you well on your vision journey.